# In praise of Gina

'Thank you so much Gina Ford. You and your books are truly heaven sent.'

'Without your books I do not know what I would have done. Your advice has meant that I have a fantastic, happy little boy and I actually look forward to the next challenge he may bring as I know where the answer to any problem lies!'

'I would like to express my gratitude for your book. It has been an absolute saviour and my best friend since I started my little boy on your routine when he was 10 weeks old. He is nearly nine months old now and everyone always says of him "what a happy contented little baby!"'

'From day one of Daisy's return home from Hospital we put her into Gina's routine and have never looked back. Everyone comments on Daisy and what an unbelievably happy and contented baby she is . . . Thank you Gina for your books and the enjoyment and confidence they have given us.'

'Gina transformed our son into the happiest, "easiest" baby, that we could have wished for. Her knowledge and professionalism is astounding; she has answers to every question – and they really work.'

'My friends tell me that it is not "normal" for a baby to be as happy and well behaved as my daughter. It certainly seems to be normal for "Gina's babies".'

'We can't recommend her highly enough to any prospective parents. We found her invaluable, and I have much to thank her for – setting us on the right path to understanding our baby's needs and being confident parents, as well as giving our son the best start in life he could get.'

# The New Contented Little Baby Book

*The secret to calm and confident parenting*

Gina Ford

Vermilion
LONDON

5 7 9 10 8 6



First published in the United Kingdom in 1999 by Vermilion
Revised edition published in 2002 by Vermilion

This edition published in 2006 by Vermilion, an imprint of
Ebury Publishing
Random House UK Ltd
Random House
20 Vauxhall Bridge Road
London SW1V 2SA

Random House Australia (Pty) Limited
20 Alfred Street, Milsons Point, Sydney,
New South Wales 2061, Australia

Random House New Zealand Limited
18 Poland Road, Glenfield, Auckland 10, New Zealand

Random House (Pty) Limited
Isle of Houghton, Corner of Boundary Road & Carse O'Gowrie,
Houghton 2198, South Africa

Random House Publishers India Private Limited
301 World Trade Tower, Hotel Intercontinental Grand Complex,
Barakhamba Lane, New Delhi 110 001, India

Random House UK Limited Reg. No. 954009
www.randomhouse.co.uk

A CIP catalogue record for this book is available from the British Library

The Random House Group Limited makes every effort to ensure that the papers used in its books are made from trees that have been legally sourced from well-managed and credibly certified forests. Our paper procurement policy can be found at: www.randomhouse.co.uk/paper/htm

ISBN: 9780091912697

FSC
Mixed Sources
Product group from well-managed forests and other controlled sources
www.fsc.org Cert no. TT-COC-2139
© 1996 Forest Stewardship Council

Printed and bound in Great Britain by
Clays Ltd, St Ives plc

Please note that conversions to imperial weights and measures are suitable equivalents and not exact.

The information given in this book should not be treated as a substitute for qualified medical advice; always consult a medical practitioner. Neither the author nor the publisher can be held responsible for any loss or claim arising out of the use, or misuse, of the suggestions made or the failure to take medical advice.

# Contents

# Acknowledgements

The first edition of *The Contented Little Baby Book* was based on my experience of working with over three hundred families around the world. I would like to say a huge thank you to you all for having so much trust and faith in my methods, and for the constant feedback that you have given me over the years as your babies have been growing up.

Keith and Janetta Hodgson deserve a very special thank you for their invaluable help in transforming my routines and feeding plans into an at-a-glance form, so making it easier reading for parents.

My family and friends have continued to be a constant support of love and encouragement. A loving thank you to William Alexander Ford, Jean and Andrew Fair, Ann Clough and Sheila Eskadale, and to dear friends Jane Revell, Carla Flodden Flint.

My agent Emma Todd has also continued to give me the most enormous support and guidance, as has my publisher Fiona MacIntyre, editor Imogen Fortes and the rest of the team at Random House. I owe them all a huge debt of gratitude for having such faith in my methods and encouraging my career as an author.

A very special thank you to my personal editors Dawn Fozzard and Gill MacCaulay who have not only helped me greatly with my books and website, but whose emotional support, encouragement and friendship are a constant comfort and inspiration to me.

Frances Howard Brown, a Princess Christian trained nanny with over 20 years experience, has given me the most enormous help and support with my website. Each month she helps deal with hundreds of questions and emails from readers of my books and members of the website. A very big thank you, also to Rory Jenkins of Embado.com whose technical skills have helped create a wonderful supportive community online, that reaches parents across five continents.

Finally, I would also like to say thank you to the thousands of parents who have taken the time to write to me since the first publication of this book seven years ago, telling me of their experiences of using the CLB routines. Your constant feedback has been very important to me, and your loving supportive messages, mean more to me than you will ever know. Special love and thanks to you all and to your contented babies.

# Foreword

## The baby book that is different

With the massive amount of information and knowledge available on raising children from birth, it is a difficult task for new parents to know where to start. If you do have some spare time after pregnancy to read about postnatal care, you will find there is no information on how to cope day by day, and nothing to help you understand the changes that will occur on a week-to-week basis in a quick and easily digestible form.

This is where Gina comes to the rescue with her hour-by-hour, week-by-week guide on how to get a baby into a sensible routine. A series of clear guides chart the changes in the needs of baby and parents, so that at a glance you can see how to cope with this new way of life, one day at a time, from week to week.

Whether you are breast-feeding or bottle-feeding, Gina takes you through a typical day, helping you manage both the baby and your time, and teaches you to understand the changes that the baby will go through. Then as the feeding needs of your baby change, she demonstrates how to start the weaning process of introducing solids, with forward-looking advice on how and why to adapt the baby's menu.

All the 300 or so babies that Gina has helped look after are a happy testament to how a routine can help. Gina uses her hands-on experience on how to get the best for your baby and uses actual examples of problems she has encountered to help the reader to understand and solve the problems they might have.

Keith Hodgson

*Father of Jake Jupiter Hodgson – born 2.1.96 – a true Gina baby, who sleeps 12 hours every night has always eaten well and is happy and content in all ways.*

# Introduction

My first book, *The Contented Little Baby Book* (first published in 1999) was based on my personal experiences of working with over 300 babies and their families in many different parts of the world. It became a bestseller and has been used, and continues to be used, by hundreds of thousands of families across five continents.

The popularity of my advice, and loyal support of the book's followers, is testimony that babies can and do thrive very successfully on routines. Unlike the old-fashioned and inflexible four-hourly routines, my routines are based upon a baby's natural feeding and sleeping rhythms, ensuring that a baby's needs are met before he gets distressed or over-tired. Most importantly, the routines can be adapted to suit the individual needs of each baby; from extensive experience, I know that all babies are different.

In the time since my first book was published, I have communicated with thousands of parents as a result of my consultancy work and through the Contented Baby website, www.contentedbaby.com. This regular and direct contact has enabled me to obtain useful feedback from parents on the Contented Little Baby (CLB) routines, which in turn has inspired me to fully revise and update my original book. The CLB routines and my core philosophy remain the same, but my advice has been expanded in response to this valuable feedback, and adapted to today's circumstances.

I am confident that this revised book will be even better at teaching you how to recognise the difference between hunger and tiredness, how to establish good feeding and sleeping patterns and how to meet all of your precious baby's needs. With help from this totally revised version of *The New Contented Little Baby Book*, becoming a parent should be a happy and deeply satisfying experience for both you and your baby. The CLB routines have worked for many thousands of parents and their contented babies, and they can work for you too.

Gina Ford

# Preparation for the birth | 1

When one talks of preparing for the birth, the first things that spring to mind are antenatal care and decorating the nursery. Both are important in their own ways. Antenatal care is of the utmost importance for a healthy pregnancy and helps to prepare you for the birth; and decorating the nursery for the new arrival is fun. While many of the antenatal classes on offer do give some advice on what is ahead after the birth, they often focus on the birth itself and overlook very practical tips, which, if offered early enough, could save parents hours of time and stress after their baby is born.

If you follow my routines from day one you should be fortunate enough to have a contented and happy baby, with some time for yourself. However, as you will see from my routines and charts, spare time is extremely limited (and, believe me, mothers who are not following a routine have even less spare time). In this short amount of time, unless you have hired help, you will have to fit in the cooking of meals, shopping, laundry etc.

By doing the following things before the baby is born you will gain many hours of free time after the birth.

- Order all your nursery equipment well in advance. Cots can sometimes take up to 12 weeks to be delivered and there are many advantages in having the big cot from the beginning (see page 3).
- Have all the bed linen, muslins and towels washed and ready for use. Make up the cot, Moses basket and pram. Prepare everything in the nursery so it is at hand the minute you get home from the hospital.

- Have the following baby essentials in stock: cotton wool, baby oil, nappies, nappy and moisturising creams, baby wipes, soft sponges, baby brush, bath oil and baby shampoo.
- Check that all the electrical equipment is working properly. Learn how the steriliser works and how to put together the feeding bottles.
- Arrange a section of work-top in the kitchen where preparation and sterilisation can be done. Ideally, it should be directly below a cupboard where all the baby's feeding equipment can be stored.
- Stock up on soap powder, cleaning materials and enough kitchen and toilet rolls to last at least six weeks.
- Prepare and freeze a large selection of healthy home-made meals for you and your husband/partner. If you are breast-feeding you should avoid the shop-bought ones that are full of additives and preservatives.
- Stock up on extra dry goods such as tea, coffee, biscuits etc; it is inevitable that you will have extra visitors the first month, and supplies will soon go down.
- Purchase birthday gifts and cards for any forthcoming birthdays. Also have a good selection of thank you cards ready to send for all the gifts you will receive.
- Get up to date with any odd jobs that need to be done in the house or garden. The last thing you need once the baby has arrived is the hassle of workmen to-ing and fro-ing.
- If breast-feeding, book your electric expressing machine well in advance; they are in big demand! Ask your midwife for advice on how to do this.

## The nursery

Like most parents, you will probably have your baby sleeping in your room with you during the night. However, I can't stress enough the importance of having the nursery ready on your return from the hospital. All too often a mother will ring me up in a complete panic asking for advice on how to get a three-month-old baby used to their own room. Many tears and much anxiety could have been avoided if the mother had got the baby used to his own room from day one. Instead, for the first few weeks, the baby dozes on and off during the early part of the evening in a car seat, then is taken to the parents' room for the last feed and the night. It is not surprising that these babies feel very abandoned when they are eventually put to sleep by themselves in an unfamiliar, dark room.

From the very beginning, you should use the nursery for nappy changing and naps. In the evening after the bath, feed and settle the baby there from 7pm to 10pm. The baby can still be transferred to your room after the last feed, to make middle-of-the-night feeding easier. But by getting your baby used to his room from the beginning, he will very quickly enjoy being there and see it as a peaceful haven, not a prison.

When my babies are very small, if they have become overtired or overstimulated, I find that they will calm down immediately when taken to their room. And by six weeks they are positively beaming when taken to their nursery for the bath and bedtime routine.

## Decoration

It is not essential to spend a fortune on decorating and furnishing the baby's room. A room with walls, windows and bed linen covered in teddy bears soon becomes very boring. Plain walls can easily be brightened up with a colourful frieze, and perhaps a matching pelmet and tie-backs; this makes it easy to adapt the room as the baby grows, but avoids the need to redecorate totally. (Another very cost-effective and fun way to liven up the room is to use sheets of children's wrapping paper as posters, which are bright and colourful – and can be changed frequently.)

## The cot

Most baby books advise that in the early days a cot is not necessary, as babies are happier in a Moses basket or small crib. I am not convinced they are happier and sleep better in these.

As I have said, I much prefer to get my babies used to their big cot from day one. By doing this, I have never encountered a problem when they outgrow the Moses basket and start to sleep the whole night in their big cot in the nursery.

When choosing a cot, it is important to remember that it will be your baby's bed for at least two or three years and should therefore be sturdy enough to withstand a bouncing toddler. Even very young babies will eventually move around their cot.

I would suggest choosing a design with flat spars instead of round ones, as pressing the head against a round spar could be quite painful for a young baby. Cot bumpers are not advised for babies less than one year old, as they can end up sleeping with their heads pressed up against the bumpers. Because body heat escapes through the top of the head, blocking it off increases the risk of overheating. This is thought to be a contributing factor in cot death.

Other points to bear in mind when choosing cots are:

- Look for two or three different base height levels.
- Drop-sides should be easy to put up and down without making a noise. Test several times.
- The cot should be large enough to accommodate a two-year-old child comfortably.
- All cots must comply with the recommendations set out by the British Standards Institute, Number BS1753. Spars must be no less than 2.5cm (1in) apart and no more than 6cm (2½ in). When the mattress is at its lowest position, the maximum distance between that and the cot top should be no more than 65cm (26in). There should be a gap of no more than 4cm (1½ in) around the edge of the mattress.
- Buy the best possible mattresses that you can afford. I have found that foam mattresses tend to sink in the middle within a few months. The type I have found to give the best support for growing babies is a 'natural cotton spring interior' type. All mattresses must comply with Safety Standards Numbers BS1877 and BS7177.

## Bedding for the cot

Everything should be 100 per cent white cotton so that it can be washed on a hot wash along with the baby's night clothes. Due to the risk of overheating or smothering, quilts and duvets are not recommended for babies under one year old. If you want a pretty matching top cover for your baby's cot, make sure it is 100 per cent cotton and not quilted with a nylon filling. For parents who are handy with a sewing machine, a considerable amount of money can be saved by making flat sheets and draw sheets out of a large cotton double bed sheet.

*Making up the cot*

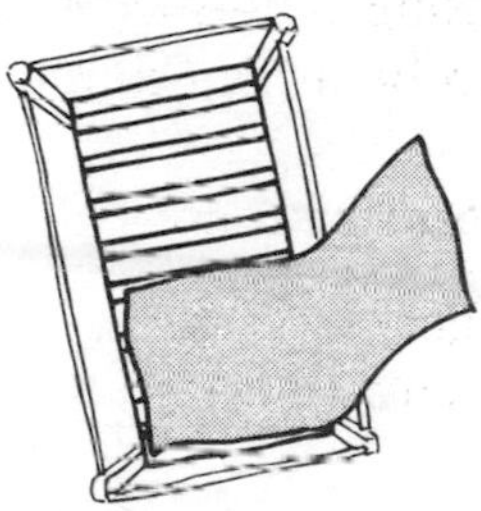

(a) Remove mattress and lay a sheet and blanket lengthways across the base of the cot.

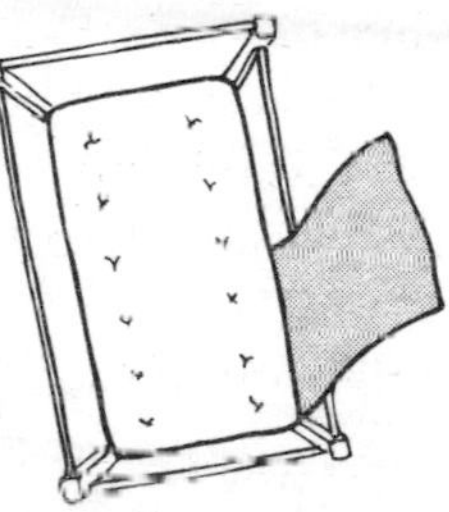

(b) Replace mattress and cover with bottom sheet.

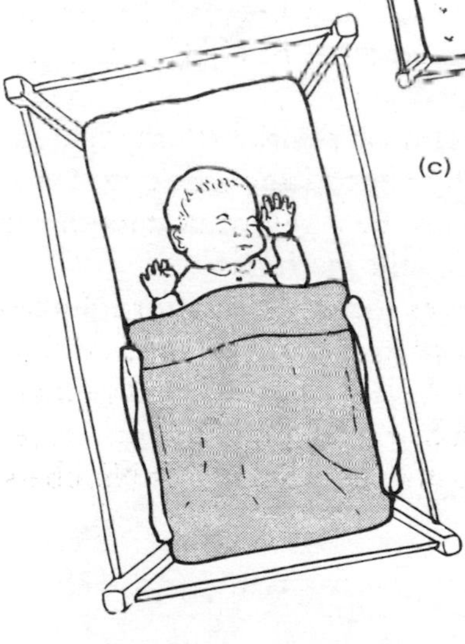

(c) Place sheet over baby and tuck in at least 15cm (6in) at the other side. Push a small, rolled-up towel down either side between the cot mattress and spars.

You will need at least the following bedding:

- Three stretch-cotton fitted bottom sheets. Choose the soft jersey-type cotton rather than the towelling type, which can very quickly become rough and worn-looking.
- Three flat, smooth cotton top sheets. Avoid flannelette, which gives off too much fluff for young babies; this can obstruct the nose and cause breathing problems.
- Three cotton, small-weave cellular blankets, plus one wool blanket for very cold nights.
- Six flat, smooth cotton pram sheets. These are small sheets that are used for prams and Moses baskets, but are also ideal as draw sheets, which you should put across the head end of the bottom sheet. This eliminates the need to remake the whole cot in the middle of the night or during naps, should your baby dribble or his nappy leak.

### Changing station

The most practical changing station is a long unit, containing drawers and a cupboard. The top should be long enough to hold both the changing mat and the top-and-tail bowl. The drawers can be used to store nightwear, underwear and muslins, and the cupboard can hold larger items, such as nappy packs.

### Wardrobe

A fitted wardrobe is a very good investment for your nursery as it enables you to keep the baby's clothes tidy and crease-free, and it will also provide valuable storage space for the many pieces of equipment that you will accumulate. If a fitted wardrobe is out of the question, try to purchase a free-standing version.

### Chair

It is essential, no matter how small your baby's room is, that you try to fit in a chair. A really sturdy comfortable chair is an absolute priority. A small two-seater bed-settee is a good choice as it can be used for both feeding and for sleeping in the baby's room. If space is limited, then choose a chair with a straight back. It should be wide enough to allow room for you and your baby as he grows, and, ideally, the arms should be wide enough to support you while breast-feeding. I would resist the temptation to buy a rocking chair, which is often sold as a nursing chair. These can prove to be dangerous as the baby becomes more mobile and may attempt to pull himself up by holding on to the chair. In the early days it can also be tempting to settle your baby by rocking him to sleep, but this is one of the main causes of a baby developing poor sleeping habits.

### Curtains

Curtains should be full-length and fully lined with black-out lining (see Useful Addresses page 232). Fix them to a track that fits flush along the top of the window. Ideally, they should have a deep matching pelmet, which is also lined with blackout lining. There should be no gaps between the sides of the curtains and the window frame; even the smallest chink of light can be enough to wake your babies earlier than 7am. For the same reason, curtain poles should be avoided as the light streams through the gap at the top. As your baby gets older, he may not settle back to sleep if woken at 5am by early morning sun in the summer, or streetlights.

When the lights are off and the curtains are closed, it should be so dark that you are unable to see your partner standing at the other side of the room. Research has also shown that the chemicals in the brain alter in the dark, conditioning the body for sleep.

### Carpeting

A fully fitted carpet is preferable to rugs, which have the potential for tripping on when you are attending to your baby in dim light. Choose a carpet that is treated with a stain-guard, and avoid very dark or bright colours, as they tend to show the dirt more easily.

### Lighting

If the main light in the nursery is not already fitted with a dimmer switch, it would be worthwhile changing it. In the early days, dimming the lights when settling the baby is a good association signal. If you are on a limited budget, purchase one of the small plug-in night-lights that fit into any normal 13-amp electrical socket.

## Baby equipment

### Moses basket or small crib

As I mentioned earlier, a Moses basket is not really essential. Even the cheapest of Moses baskets and a stand can cost over £50, which is quite a lot of money for something unessential that your baby will outgrow within six weeks. However, if you live in a very large house or plan to travel in the first few weeks, it may be useful. If your budget is limited, try to borrow one from a friend and buy a new mattress.

A crib is a small version of a big cot. Certainly, it is longer than a Moses basket, but not really any more practical. Because we now put our babies to sleep on their backs, these narrow cribs create a problem for small babies. They can wake themselves up several times a night because the cribs are not wide enough for them to sleep with their arms stretched out fully, and they get their hands caught between the spars.

If you do decide to use either of the above for a short period, you will need the following bedding:

- Three fixed, stretch cotton bottom sheets. Choose the soft, smooth jersey-type cotton.
- Six smooth cotton flat pram sheets, to be used as top sheets and later as draw sheets on the big cot.
- Four cotton, cellular close-weave pram blankets.
- A dozen muslins to be placed across the top of the basket or crib to catch dribbles.

## Pram

The traditional pram is very expensive and not really appropriate to modern-day living. Most parents find it more practical to choose one of the other smaller types of transport available now. When choosing a pram, carry-cot or buggy, it is important to take into consideration where you live and your lifestyle. For example, if you have to drive to the nearest shops, it is important to choose a buggy that is easy to put up and down and not too heavy for constant lifting in and out of the car boot. There are now some very lightweight buggies on the market that recline flat for a newborn baby, and come with hood and apron to give the baby some protection in cold weather.

Another popular choice with parents is a 'three-in-one', which is a transporter that can be used with a carry-cot in the early days and later with a buggy type seat. This can be a very good choice if you live in a quieter area and can walk to the local shops. The third choice is a heavier weight version of the light buggy; it also reclines flat for a newborn and usually comes with a mattress.

If you are likely to be using your pram or buggy in a town area, or in shops with narrow spaces (for example, aisles in supermarkets), swivel wheels are a godsend. They make turning the buggy or pram round corners effortless compared to those with set wheels.

Whichever type you choose, you should practise putting it up and down several times, and try lifting it on to a surface in the shop to get an idea of how easy it is going to be to lift into the boot.

The following guidelines should also be followed when purchasing a pram, carry-cot or buggy:

- It should be fitted with good strong safety straps that go over the baby's shoulders as well as around the waist, and have an easy-to-operate brake.
- Make sure it has a hood and apron to protect the baby in colder weather.
- Buy all the extras at the same time: sun canopy, rain cover,

cosytoes cover, head support cushion and shopping tray or bag. Models often change in design and sometimes dimension, and if you wait till the following season, the items you require might not fit or match.
- Try pushing it around the shop to check if the handle height is a comfortable level; also observe how easy it is to get in and out of doorways and round corners.

### Car seat

You will need to have a car seat to bring your baby home from hospital. A midwife often accompanies parents to the car to check that all is in order as mother and baby are discharged. A baby car seat should always be used, even on short journeys. Never be tempted to travel holding your baby in your arms as, in the event of a collision or emergency stop, it would be impossible to keep hold of your baby. Car seats should not be fitted to the front passenger seat if the car has airbags, unless these have been adequately disabled. In general, choose the best you can afford, and preferably ones that come with clear fitting instructions.

Other things to look for include:

- A seat with large side wings, which offer more protection in a side-impact collision.
- A one-pull harness, which will make it much easier to adjust the seat to your baby's clothing.
- The buckle should be easy to open and close, but not easy enough for a child to open.
- The availability of extra accessories, such as a head support pillow or replacement cover.

### Baby bath

A baby bath is another item that is not essential. Like the Moses basket, babies outgrow the small bath very quickly. A newborn baby can be bathed in the hand basin to begin with, or even in a big bath using one of the several types of bath seats that are available for tiny babies. These allow the baby to lie, supported and on a slight slope, leaving the mother with both hands free to wash the baby.

If you would feel more confident with a special baby bath, the one I would recommend is designed to fit across a big bath. It makes filling and emptying much easier, unlike the traditional baby bath that sits on a stand, and has to be filled and emptied using a bucket. Another design is a bath that is incorporated in a changing station. I have found these totally impractical because, as you lift the baby out of the bath, you have to manoeuvre the lid, which doubles as the changing table, down over the top of the bath before you can put the baby on it to dry and dress him. They are also very difficult to empty; I found I always had to tip the whole thing on its side to drain the water out completely. This usually ended up with all the items stored below toppling out on to the floor. These bath/changing stations are very expensive and I would discourage anyone from buying them.

## Changing mat

It is worthwhile buying two changing mats. Choose easy-clean plastic with well-padded sides. In the early days it is best to lay a hand towel on the top, as very young babies hate to be laid down on anything cold.

## Baby monitor

This is an important piece of equipment, so don't skimp when buying it. There are generally two types to choose from, plug-in and mobile, but I would advise you to look at the mobile version, which allows you to move freely around the house, including areas such as the bathroom, which does not have an electrical socket for the plug-in version.

When choosing a baby monitor, look for the following features:

- A visual light display as well as sound, which allows you to monitor your baby even with the volume turned down.

- Monitors work using radio channels, so choose a model with two channels, which allows you to switch channels if there is interference.
- A rechargeable model is more expensive initially, but the saving on batteries will make it cheaper in the long run.
- A low-battery indicator and an out-of-range indicator.

### Baby sling

Some parents swear by this method of moving around with their babies. I never use one as I find it too big a strain on my back to carry a baby around like this for any length of time. Very small babies are also inclined to go straight to sleep the minute you hold them close to your chest, which defeats the whole purpose of my routines – i.e. keeping the baby awake at certain times of the day, and teaching the baby the right associations of going to sleep on his own. I do think that as babies get bigger, slings are a very useful way for parents to carry them around, especially when the baby is old enough to face forward.

If you feel a sling would be useful, here are some guidelines to observe when choosing one:

- The sling must have safety tabs to ensure it cannot come undone.
- It must provide your baby with enough head and neck support; some come with a detachable cushion that gives extra support for very young babies.
- It should offer the choice of baby facing in or outwards and have a seat with an adjustable height position.
- It should be made of strong, washable fabric with comfortable, padded shoulder straps.
- I would certainly recommend trying it on in the shop and putting a baby into it – one size does not fit all!

### Baby chair

While many parents use the car seat in the house for their baby to sit in during the day, if your budget will stretch to it having a second seat for your baby can be a great bonus as it saves having to move seats from room to room.

Baby seats come in different styles. Some chairs are rigid with adjustable seat positions and a base that can either remain stable or be set to rocking mode. Another type is known as a 'bouncy chair'. This type is made of a lightweight frame covered in fabric and is designed to bounce as the baby moves. I have found them to be very popular with babies over two months, but they can make tiny babies feel insecure. Whatever type of chair you choose, make sure your baby is securely strapped in and never left unattended. Also, always place the baby on the floor when in a seat; never be tempted to leave him on a table or work-top, as the movement of the baby can easily shift the chair to the edge.

Here are some further guidelines:

- The frame and base should be firm and sturdy, and fitted with a strong safety strap.
- Choose one with an easily removable and washable cover.
- Buy a head support cushion for tiny babies.

### Playpen

Playpens are frowned upon by some 'baby experts', who feel they hinder a baby's natural instinct to explore. My own feeling is that, while babies should never be left for long periods in a playpen, they can be very useful for ensuring your child is safe when you are preparing lunch or need to answer the door. If you do decide to use a playpen, I would recommend getting your baby used to it from a young age. A travel cot can be used as a playpen but, if you have the space, I would recommend the square wooden type, which is larger and would enable your baby to pull himself up and move around. Whichever sort you choose, make sure it is situated out of reach of hazards such as radiators, curtains and trailing flexes. Never hang toys on pieces of string or cord in the playpen, as these could prove fatal if your baby were to get tangled up.

Important points to look for when choosing a playpen are:

- Make sure it has a fixed floor so that your baby cannot move it.
- Check that there are no sharp metal hinges or catches on which your baby could harm himself.
- If choosing a mesh-type playpen or travel cot, make sure that the mesh is strong enough to prevent your baby pushing small toys through and making a hole big enough to trap his hand or fingers.

## Equipment needed for breast-feeding

### Nursing bra

These are bras made with specially designeds that can either be unhooked or unzipped to make breast-feeding easier. It is important that whatever style of bra you choose fits well. A good nursing bra should preferably be made of cotton for comfort, have wide, adjustable shoulder straps to help support your breasts, and should not press tightly against the nipples as this can be a cause of blocked milk ducts. I would suggest buying two before the birth. If they prove comfortable after your milk has come in, a further two can be purchased.

### Breast pads

In the early days you will use a lot of breast pads, as they need to be changed every time your baby feeds. Many mothers prefer the round ones, contoured to fit the breasts. You may need to experiment with different brands, but sometimes the more expensive ones offer better absorbency, so can work out better value in the long run.

### Nursing pillow

These pillows are shaped to fit around a mother's waist, bringing small babies up to the perfect height for breast-feeding. They can also be used for propping babies up and make an excellent back support for older babies who are learning to sit up. If you decide to invest in one, make sure it has a removable, machine-washable cover.

### Nipple cream and sprays

These are designed to care for the breasts and help relieve any pain caused by breast-feeding. The main cause of pain, however, is poor positioning of the baby on the breast. If you experience pain either during or after feeding, it would be wise to consult your health visitor or breast-feeding counsellor for advice before purchasing a cream or spray. No other special creams or soaps are recommended when breast-feeding. Simply wash your breasts twice a day with plain water and after each feed. The nipples should be rubbed with a little breast milk and allowed to airdry.

### Electric expressing machine

I am convinced that one of the reasons the majority of mothers I advise are successful at breast-feeding is because I encourage the use of an electric expressing machine. In the very early days when you are producing more milk than your baby may need (especially first thing in the morning), this can be expressed using one of these powerful machines. The expressed milk can then be stored in the fridge or freezer and used as a top-up later in the day when you are becoming tired and your milk supply may be low. This, I believe, is one of the main reasons why so many babies are restless and will not settle after their bath in the evening. If you want to breast-feed and quickly establish your baby in a routine, an electric breast pump will be a big asset. Do not be tempted by one of the smaller hand versions, which can be so inefficient as to put many women off expressing at all.

### Freezer bags

Expressed milk can be stored in the fridge for up to 24 hours, or in the freezer for one month. Specially designed, pre-sterilised bags are an ideal way to store expressed breast milk and are available from chemists or baby departments in the larger stores.

**Feeding bottles**

Most breast-feeding counsellors are against newborn babies being given a bottle, even of expressed milk. They claim that it creates nipple confusion, reducing the baby's desire to suck on the breast, leading in turn to poor milk supply and the mother giving up breast-feeding altogether. My own view is that the majority of women give up breast-feeding because they are totally exhausted with 'demand feeding', often several times a night. I advise giving babies a bottle of either expressed milk or formula milk from the first week and introducing it by the fourth week at the latest. This one bottle can be given either last thing in the evening or during the night by someone other than the mother, thereby allowing the mother to sleep for several hours at a stretch. This, in turn, is likely to make her more able to cope with breast-feeding. I have never had a problem with a baby rejecting the mother's breast or becoming confused between nipple and teat, but this could happen if, in the early days, a baby was offered more than one bottle a day. Other good reasons for getting your baby used to a bottle are: firstly, it gives you some flexibility; secondly, the problem of later introducing bottles to an exclusively breast-fed baby doesn't arise; and thirdly, it gives the baby's father a wonderful opportunity to become more involved.

There are many types of bottle available, all claiming to be the best. From experience, the make I have liked the best is the wide-necked design by Avent. The wide neck makes cleaning and filling easier and I support their claim that the design of the teat reduces the amount of wind that gets into a baby's stomach. I suggest that you start off by using a slow-flow teat, which will encourage your baby to work as hard drinking milk from a bottle as when breast-feeding. For advice on sterilising equipment required, please refer to the next section.

# Equipment needed for bottle-feeding

### Feeding bottles

For the reasons already mentioned, I would strongly advise buying the wide-necked bottles described above. If your baby is likely to take all his milk from a bottle, it is important that the risk of developing colic or wind is kept to a minimum. When called upon to help a baby with colic, I often see an immediate improvement simply by switching to these wide-necked bottles. The teat is designed to be flexible and it allows the baby to suckle as he would at the breast. The wide-necked bottles, in time, can also be adapted to become feeding beakers with soft spouts and handles. If your baby is being exclusively bottle-fed, I would advise that you start off with five 240ml (8oz) bottles and three 120ml (4oz) bottles.

### Teats

Most feeding bottles come with a slow-flow teat designed to meet the needs of newborns. By eight weeks I have found that most babies feed better from a medium-flow teat and it is worthwhile stocking up on these extra teats from the beginning.

### Bottle brush

Proper and thorough cleaning of your baby's bottles is of the utmost importance. Try to choose a brush with an extra-long plastic handle, which will allow more force to be put into cleaning the bottles.

### Teat brush

Most mothers find that the easiest way to clean a teat is by using their forefinger. However, if you have extra-long nails, it may be worthwhile investing in one of these brushes, although they too can damage the hole of the teat, resulting in the need to replace the teats more frequently. Short nails are probably the answer!

### Washing-up bowl

It is easier to organise and keep track of what is sterilised if all the dirty bottles are washed and sterilised at the same time. You will need somewhere to put the rinsed-out bottles and teats until they are ready to be sterilised, and a large stainless steel or plastic bowl can be used for this purpose, preferably with a lid.

### Steriliser

Whether breast- or bottle-feeding, it is essential that all bottles and expressing equipment be sterilised properly. There are three main methods of sterilisation: boiling equipment for 10 minutes in a large pan; soaking equipment in a sterilising solution for two hours and rinsing with boiling water; or using an electric steam steriliser. From experience, the easiest, fastest and most effective method is the steam steriliser, and it is well worth making this investment. A word of caution – don't be tempted to purchase a microwave version. This type of unit not only holds fewer bottles, but it becomes a complete nuisance when you have to remove it to use the microwave for other purposes.

### Kettle

Obviously essential for making up feeds, so your kettle should be efficient and of sufficient size. If, for personal reasons, you decide to formula-feed right from the beginning you will spend a lot of time in the first year making up feeds. You might, therefore, consider investing in an extra kettle. The water for the formula needs to be fresh, boiled just once and cooled before the powder is added. If someone comes along to make a cup of tea while you are waiting for your water to cool, you'll have to start all over again. This can drive you crazy so an extra kettle just for the baby's water is often a wise investment. If you're expecting twins, it is essential.

### Electric bottle-warmer

An electric bottle-warmer is not essential, as formula can be heated by standing the bottle in a jug of boiling water. It can, however, be very useful in the nursery for the 6–6.30pm feed as it saves having to transport a jug of boiling water from room to room. There is a design that includes a bowl which fits on top, and this can be used for keeping food warm once your baby starts on solids.

### Bottle insulator

This is a special type of Thermos that is designed to keep bottles of boiled water warm. It can be very useful when travelling, or for making up night feeds quickly. When buying a bottle insulator, I would also recommend purchasing a small, plastic, three-sectioned container. Each section can then hold the required amount of formula for three different feeds, which avoids having to carry the tin of formula on days out or for the night feed.

## Clothes for the newborn

The range of babywear available in the shops is both delightful and bewildering. While it can be fun choosing garments for your baby, I would urge you to approach this particular area with caution. Newborn babies grow at an alarming rate and will outgrow most of their first-size clothes by the first month, unless they were very small at birth. Although it is important to have enough clothes to allow for frequent changing, if you have too many, most will never get worn. You will need to renew your baby's wardrobe at least three times in the first year, and even if you stick to the cheaper ranges, it will still be a costly business. I would advise you to buy only the basics before your baby arrives. You may receive clothing as gifts when your baby arrives and you will have plenty of opportunity for clothes shopping during the first year.

When choosing clothes for the first month, don't be tempted by brightly coloured underwear or sleepwear. Newborn babies have a tendency to leak from both ends and it is impossible to remove stains by washing at anything less than 60°C. Brightly coloured garments will soon lose their appearance if frequently washed at this temperature, so stick to white, and leave the brighter colours for the outer garments.

In general, keep clothing simple during the first month. Dressing your baby in little white vests and white baby-grows in the early days makes washing so much easier when you can stick everything into the same load. If possible, invest in a tumble-dryer: it is well worth the expense and means that you do not have to worry about ironing if you remove everything from the dryer the minute it is dry. Listed below are the basic items you will need for the first couple of months. Until your baby arrives, I would advise against the removal of packaging or tags, so the items can be exchanged if your baby is either larger or smaller than expected.

| | | | |
|---|---|---|---|
| Vests | 6–8 | Socks | 2–3 pairs |
| Nightdresses or sleepsuits | 4–6 | Hats | 2 |
| Day outfits | 4–6 | Mittens | 2 pairs |
| Cardigans | 2–3 | Shawl | 3 |
| Snowsuit for a winter baby | 1 | Jacket | 1 |

### Vests

A newborn baby would normally wear a vest in both winter and summer, except in very hot weather. The best fabric next to a baby's skin is 100 per cent cotton, and if you want your beautiful layette to retain its appearance after numerous hot washes, stick to plain white, or white with a pale colour pattern. The best style of vest to buy is a 'body suit', which fastens under your baby's legs, has short sleeves and an envelope-style neckline for easy dressing.

### Nightwear

The most common type of sleepwear is an all-in-one suit or baby-grow. They are snug and save time on laundry, but they can be awkward if you have to struggle to get your otherwise settled baby out of one to change his nappy. For this reason, some mothers prefer nightdresses. As with vests, 100 per cent cotton is best, and the simpler the design the better. Avoid anything with ties at the neck, and if there are ties at the bottom, remove them as they could get caught around your baby's feet.

### Day outfits

During the first couple of months, the easiest thing to dress your baby in will be baby-grows, which usually come in packs of two or three. If possible, try to buy pure cotton and choose a style that opens up either across the back or inside the legs, to ensure you don't need to undress your baby fully at nappy change. Dungaree-style clothes, without feet and with matching T-shirts, are also useful. They will last a bit longer as your baby grows, and the tops can be interchanged if your baby dribbles a lot. Choose styles in soft velour for very young babies, rather than stiff cotton or denim.

### Cardigans

If your baby is born in the summer, you could probably get away with just two cardigans, ideally in cotton. With a winter baby, it would be best to have at least three cardigans, preferably wool. As long as your baby has cotton garments next to his skin, there should be no cause for irritation, and the simpler the design the better.

### Socks

Simple socks in cotton or wool are the most practical for new babies. Fancy styles with ribbons should be avoided, as should any type of shoe, however cute, as they could harm your baby's soft bones.

### Hats

In the summer, it is important that you buy a cotton hat with a brim to protect your baby's head and face from the sun. Ideally, the brim should go right round the back of the neck. In spring and autumn, knitted cotton hats are adequate on cooler days. During the winter, or on very cold days, I would suggest a warm wool or fleece hat. Many of these are lined with cotton, but if not, a thin cotton hat can be worn underneath to protect sensitive skin.

### Mittens

Small babies do not like to have their hands covered up, as they use them extensively to touch, feel and explore everything in close contact. If, however, your baby has sharp nails or tends to scratch, you could try the fine cotton mitts made for this purpose. In very cold weather use woollen or fleece mitts, but again, put cotton ones underneath if your baby has sensitive skin.

### Shawl

I firmly believe that during the first few weeks all babies sleep better when swaddled. Whether you choose a blanket or shawl to swaddle, it should always be made of lightweight pure cotton that has a slight stretch to it. To avoid overheating, always swaddle your baby in a single layer, and when sleeping swaddled, reduce the number of blankets on the cot. It is, however, important that by six weeks you start to get your baby used to being half-swaddled, under the arms. Cot death rates peak between two and four months and overheating is thought to be a major factor. Always check that you are not putting too many layers on and that the temperature of the room remains between 16 and 20°C, as recommended by the Foundation for the Study of Infant Deaths.

### Snowsuit

When choosing snowsuits for your baby, always buy at least two sizes too big, as this allows plenty of room for growth.

*How to swaddle your baby*

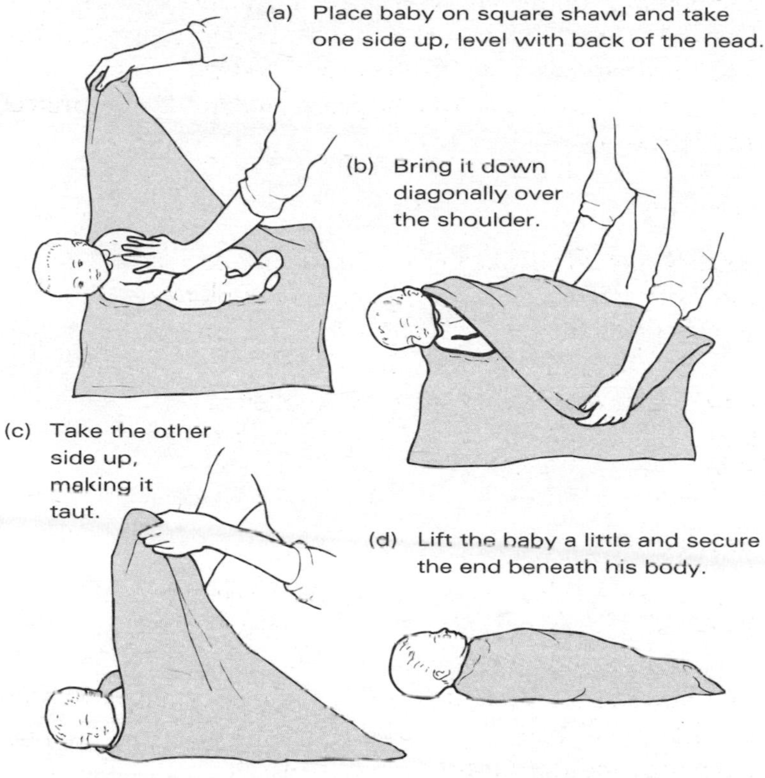


Avoid fancy designs with fur around the hood or dangling toggles, opting instead for one in an easy-care washable fabric. For tiny babies, poppers may be preferable to a zip, which can dig into the chin.

### Jacket

A lightweight jacket can be useful for babies born at any time of the year. In summer it can be worn on chilly days, and in winter on milder ones. As with the snowsuits, choose one in a simple design in a washable fabric.

# Your baby's laundry

Having spent a considerable amount of time and money on your baby's wardrobe, it is well worth the effort to be very fussy about caring for it. Because young babies grow out of their clothes so quickly, it should be possible, with good laundering, to pass them on to any brother or sister that follows.

The following guidelines will help keep your baby's laundry in tiptop condition:

- Laundry should be sorted into different-coloured lots.
- Bedding, muslins and bibs need to be washed on a very hot wash to get rid of bacteria caused by milk stains and to eliminate the house dust mite, which can trigger allergies in very young babies.
- Load the washing machine no more than two-thirds full so that the clothes are rinsed thoroughly.
- Stains should always be treated before washing.

### Whites: 60°—90°C

Anything that is stained should be soaked overnight in a cold solution of Napisan, then washed at 60°C. Everything should be 100 per cent cotton, and bibs or towels with a coloured trim should have been tested for colour-run by washing separately for the first few washes. Sheets, muslins, vests, bibs, socks and white sleepsuits and nighties can also go in at 60°C if they are not very dirty. If they have not been soaked and are very dirty, they should go in a 90°C wash. Towels and face-cloths should be washed and dried together, and separate from other clothes, to avoid bobbling.

### Light colours: 40°C

Most day clothes need only a very quick wash in the wool or delicate cycle. Anything stained should be soaked first overnight in cold water and Napisan, and rinsed before washing.

### Dark colours: 30°C or handwash

Any dark outfits must be washed separately from the light colours even if they do not run; to mix the two will only result in the lighter colours taking on a grey tinge. Anything stained should be soaked first overnight in cold water and soap powder.

### Woollens or delicates: handwash

Even if the label says 'machine wash' it is better to handwash using a very small amount of Filetti (baby soap powder) mixed with lukewarm water. Always squeeze the garment gently in the water when washing and rinsing; never wring, twist or allow a delicate garment to hang down. Rinse thoroughly in cold running water, gently squeeze out excess water, then roll in a clean, dry, white towel for a few hours. Finally, gently pull into shape and either dry flat or hang across a drying screen. Never hang up woollens from the bottom.

### Use of the tumble-dryer

Towels, bibs, fitted cot sheets and blankets can be tumble-dried, but flat cotton sheets should be dried so that they are slightly damp for easier and smoother ironing. Avoid drying towels and clothes together as it causes bobbling. Remove all clothes from the dryer and fold them as soon as possible to avoid creasing, and ensure that all clothes are properly aired.

### Corduroy and dark clothes

To avoid fading and shadowing, dry these on the cool cycle for no more than 15 minutes. Then pull the clothes into shape and hang them up on hangers to dry. In this way they may not need to be ironed.

### Ironing

Flat cot sheets and draw sheets should be ironed slightly damp for a smooth finish. Light-coloured outfits should be ironed using the water spray, and dark colours must be ironed on the inside with a very cool iron. Knitwear should be pressed with a muslin cloth. Ensure that all labels are ironed flat.

# Why follow a routine? 2

Six years have passed since I first typed the four words 'why follow a routine?'. Little did I know then the controversy those four simple words would create. But here I am, six years later, explaining again why I think routine is important. I must stress that my views have not changed one little bit from when I wrote my first book. I personally believe that the majority of babies thrive and are happier in a routine. But I certainly realise and respect that following a routine is not a choice for all parents.

There is already so much advice out there for 'baby-led parenting'; therefore, the advice I give in my books is for those parents who believe that they and their baby will be happier in a routine. I assume that one of the reasons you are reading this book is that you already have a certain level of structure in your life, and that you believe you will cope with your baby better by following some sort of routine. If this is the case then I can assure you that following Contented Little Baby routines will most certainly benefit both you and your baby. They are followed successfully by hundreds of thousands of parents around the world. Follow your own instinct as a parent as to what works best for you and your baby; use the routines and advice in this book as tools to help you be the parents that you want to be.

## Why the CLB routines are different

During the years that I worked as a maternity nurse I read hundreds of books on child care, but I have also had the most unique privilege of working personally with over 300 families around the world. It is because of these parents and their beautiful babies that I feel I am able to share with you so much of what I have learned, which I hope will help you overcome many of the everyday practicalities of parenting.

As a maternity nurse I would arrive at a home a few days after the birth, and live with the family 24/7 for periods of between 3–5 days, or sometimes several weeks to six months. While the media make much of the fact that many of my clients were rich and famous, I can assure you that the majority of families I helped were not. They often had to get outside help for health issues, family bereavement or other personal circumstances. Whether they lived in a mansion with 20 bedrooms or a flat with only one bedroom, were a rock or movie star, a struggling actor, high-profile banker or teacher, these parents all had one thing in common – they each wanted to ensure that their baby was happy and contented, and that they could somehow manage to meet all of their baby's needs as well as cope with the demanding lives that they led.

The leading child care books at that time all endorsed baby-led parenting and claimed that it was impossible to put a small baby into a routine. The implication was that if parents were even to attempt to put their baby in a routine they could seriously damage the child's health.

In my first book I said that, having successfully spent many years teaching parents how to put their newborns into a routine that results in a happy, thriving, contented baby, I can only assume that the authors of these books have not personally worked with enough babies to know this is possible. The fact that *The Contented Little Baby Book* became a runaway bestseller through personal recommendation is proof enough that the statement I made in my first edition in 1999 has been proved true.

Parents who have properly read the book, the routines and the advice I give, can testify that the CLB routines do really work. Unlike old-fashioned four-hourly feeding they do not involve leaving a baby to yell until a feed is due, or leaving him to cry himself to sleep for lengthy periods. While establishing a routine is often very hard work and requires a lot of sacrifices on the part of the parents, hundreds of thousands of parents around the world will testify that it is worth it because they quickly learn how to meet the needs of their babies so that any distress is kept to a minimum.

## Benefits for your baby

The reason that the CLB routines are different from traditional four-hourly routines is that they are created to meet the natural sleep and feeding needs of all healthy normal babies. They also allow for the fact that some babies need more sleep than others, and that some may be able to go longer between feeds than others. The aim of the routines is not to push your baby through the night without a feed, but to ensure that by structuring the feeding and sleeping during the day, your baby's night-time waking will be kept to a minimum. He will wake and feed quickly before settling back to sleep. The routines also ensure that once your baby is capable of going one longer spell between feeds, this will happen in the middle of the night, not during the day. The basis of these routines evolved over many years of observing babies in my care. Some babies would develop a feeding pattern very quickly with little prompting, while others would be difficult to feed and settle for many weeks.

The main observations that I made from babies who settled quickly into a pattern were:

- The parents had a positive approach, wanted a routine and tried to keep the first couple of weeks as calm as possible.
- Handling of the baby by visitors was kept to a minimum so that the baby felt relaxed and secure in his new surroundings, (especially important when the baby is first brought home from hospital).
- The baby always had regular sleep times in the same place in a dark room or his nursery between 7pm and 7am, and, whenever possible, main naps during the day were also taken there.

- The baby was kept awake for a short spell after the daytime feeds.
- When he was awake, and had been well fed and winded, he was then stimulated and played with for short periods.
- A bedtime routine was established from day one. He would be bathed at the same time every evening, then fed and settled in a dark room. If the baby did not settle, the parents would ensure that they kept things as quiet as possible and continued to comfort him in a dimly lit room until he did eventually settle.

## Benefits for you

One of the most stressful things any parent has to endure is to listen to their baby crying, particularly if the crying goes on for any length of time and all attempts to calm the baby fail. By following the CLB routines you will soon learn the signs of hunger, tiredness, boredom or indeed many of the other reasons that cause young babies to get upset. The fact that you are able to understand his needs and meet them quickly and confidently will leave both you and your baby calm and reassured, and avoid unnecessary crying. The common situation of fretful baby and fraught parents is avoided.

The other big plus for parents following my routines is that they have free time in the evening, to relax and enjoy each other's company. This is not usually possible for parents who follow baby-led parenting, as any attachment parenting website will show the early evening is a time when these babies are often particularly fretful and require endless rocking and patting to try and keep them calm.

## Other approaches

The routines and advice in this book evolved over many years. During my time as a maternity nurse I tried and tested various ways of establishing breast-feeding and healthy sleep habits. Before I further expand on why I believe that my methods are so successful, I will briefly discuss the other methods I have had experience with over the years, which I hope will give you an insight into why I believe that the CLB routines can be of great benefit to many parents and their babies.

### Strict four-hourly feeding routine

This routine evolved when hospital birth took over from home birth several decades ago and women would stay in the maternity unit for up to 10–14 days. Their babies were bought to them from the nursery every four hours and given a strict 10–15 minutes on each breast before being returned to the nursery. Although such routines are more associated with our grandmothers' generation, there are still parents nowadays who believe that babies can be slotted into them. During my early years of working as a maternity nurse I did work with some families that adopted these routines, and for some babies they did succeed, particularly if they were formula-fed.

However, I did find that trying to establish breast-feeding with a strict four-hourly feeding schedule, where feeds were limited to a strict 10–15 minutes on each breast, did not work for the majority of babies. The mother, believing that the reason her baby was not managing to stick to the schedule was because she was not producing enough milk, would very early be pressured to introduce top-up feeds of formula in order to get the baby to feed at the right times according to the routines. I would be a multimillionaire if I had a pound for every granny who has said to me, 'My milk dried up the minute I left the hospital.' The reality was that, due to rigid routines and restricted timing of feeds, the mother's milk had started to dry up long before she left the hospital. The trend for bottle-feeding became well established in the 1950s and 1960s, with many mothers not even attempting to breast-feed. This trend continued well into the 1970s. Then, as research started to unearth more and more information regarding the health benefits of breast-feeding, the trend started to swing back again. Mothers were told not to restrict feeds and to allow their babies to feed for as long as was needed to satisfy the baby's hunger.

It is important that you understand the CLB routines are not about strict four-hourly feeding schedules. It could be many weeks before a four-hourly feeding pattern can emerge, and I would urge you not to be pressured into it, however keen you are to establish a routine. The main reasons four-hourly feeding can fail are:

- Six feeds a day in the early days are usually not enough to stimulate a good milk supply.
- Babies need to feed little and often in the early days; restricting feeding to six feeds may lead to your baby being short of his daily intake.
- Babies between one week and six weeks usually need at least 30 minutes to reach the hind milk.
- Hind milk is at least three times higher in fat content than fore milk, and is essential for satisfying your baby's hunger.

### Demand feeding

Although I did look after some babies that were put into a strict four-hourly feeding routine from birth, much of my experience in the early days of my career was with babies who were being fed on demand.

The advice given then is the same nowadays. Mothers are encouraged to let their babies take the lead, allowing their babies to feed as often and for as long as they want. This method, like the four-hourly method of feeding, did succeed for some babies, but for a huge number that I was asked to help it did not work. One thing that became obvious very early in my experience is that, quite simply, many newborn babies do not demand to be fed. This is particularly true of low-birth-weight babies and twins. That is my main objection to demand feeding. If you had had the experience of sitting by the bedside of a baby only days old fighting for his life because he has become seriously dehydrated through not being fed enough, you would probably feel the same way. Dehydration is a very serious problem amongst newborn babies and one that many new parents are now aware of.

The production of breast milk works on a supply and demand basis, so babies who are allowed to sleep for long periods between feeds are not put to the breast often enough in a 24-hour period to signal the breasts to make enough milk. Mothers are lulled into a false sense of security that they have a baby who is easy and sleeps well.

In fact, what they have is a very sleepy baby who normally, 2–3 weeks down the line, will start waking up more often and demanding more milk than the mother is producing. A pattern quickly emerges of the baby having to feed every couple of hours, day and night, in order to have his daily nutritional needs met.

The current advice is that this pattern is normal and that the baby will sort itself out, but mothers are not told that with some babies it may take months! Sometimes a pattern does occur where the baby will go longer between feeds. But this is often one where the baby is feeding so much in the night that when he does wake up for feeds during the day, they tend to be short, small feeds. This leads to a vicious circle of the baby needing to feed more in the night to satisfy his daily needs. The mother then becomes exhausted from several night-time wakings and not managing to rest enough during the day. This exhaustion can often lead to some or all of the following problems:

- Exhaustion and stress reduce the mother's milk supply, increasing the baby's need to feed little and often.
- Babies who continue to need to feed 10–12 times a day after the first week often become so exhausted from lack of quality sleep that they become even more tired, and feed for shorter and shorter periods at each feed.
- Exhaustion can lead to the mother being too tired to concentrate properly on positioning the baby correctly on the breast for any length of time.
- Poor positioning on the breast is the main reason for painful, and often cracked and bleeding nipples, which again reduces how well the baby feeds at the breast.

- A sleepy baby left too long between feeds in the early days reduces the mother's chances of building up a good milk supply.

Another reason I am so opposed to the term 'demand feeding' is that it is often taken too literally. Every time the baby cries it is fed and mothers are not taught to look for other reasons why the baby may be crying, overstimulation or overtiredness, for example.

Of course, all babies must be fed if they are hungry; no baby should be left to cry for a feed or kept to a strict timetable if he is genuinely hungry. But in my experience, and if research on sleeping problems in this country is anything to go by, a huge number of demand-fed babies do not automatically fall into a healthy sleeping pattern months down the line. Many continue to wake up and feed little and often, long after a time when they are capable of going a longer spell in the night. Another problem is that babies who continue to feed little and often invariably end up being fed to sleep. This creates a whole other set of sleeping problems, where they have learnt the wrong sleep associations and cannot get to sleep without being fed.

Whether you are the parent of a newborn baby or an older baby I would urge you not even to attempt to start the routines until you have read and understood Chapters 3 and 4 on feeding and sleeping in the first year. Because CLB routines are not like the old-fashioned four-hourly routines, it is not just a case of reading a routine in Chapter 6 and trying to fit your baby's feeding and sleeping into the times I suggest. The CLB routines change 10 times during the first year. The times given for feeding and sleeping in each set of the routines are approximate guidelines for your baby's age, not rigid rules. You need to understand the principles behind the routines so that you can make slight adjustments to ensure that your baby's individual needs are being met.

# Your questions answered

**Q I am six months pregnant and, like many new mothers-to-be, I am concerned about how I am going to cope with the sleepless nights. My antenatal class stresses the importance of demand feeding, that new babies should be fed when they need it and that I should not attempt a routine in the early days. I am concerned that if I try to follow your routines, I may be denying my baby food when he is really hungry.**

A The CLB routines are not about denying babies a feed when they are really hungry. Quite the opposite. My main concern about demand feeding with very young babies is that a great many babies do not demand to be fed in the very early days. This can lead to many serious problems, the main one being that a baby who is not feeding from the breast will not stimulate the breast to produce enough milk. We therefore arrive at the situation, three or four weeks down the line, where a mother is trying to feed her baby and not producing enough milk. A vicious circle then evolves where the mother is feeding the baby every 1–2 hours, night and day, to try to satisfy his needs – but by this time, exhaustion has set in. This is one of the main reasons why the milk supply decreases and women find they have to stop breast-feeding.

In the very early days I always advise a mother to assume that, if the baby is crying, then hunger is possibly the main reason why, and the baby should be fed. However, I do stress that if a baby is continually crying and unhappy, then you should also look for reasons why the baby cannot last the three hours between feeds. Often the baby has not been latched on properly to the breast and, while he may appear to be constantly sucking for up to an hour, much of the time he is not actually drinking well. This is why mothers who are breast-feeding and finding that their baby is not going happily for 2–3 hours between feeds should always seek advice from an experienced breast-feeding counsellor. Any healthy baby weighing more than 2.7kg (6lbs) at birth should manage to go three hours between feeds – that is, three hours from the beginning of a feed to the beginning of the next feed. This will only happen if the baby receives enough milk to satisfy his needs.

**Q Do I really have to wake my newborn baby up to feed him? He wants to sleep all the time and I am tempted to leave him.**

**A** I do understand. It is a great temptation when you are tired from the birth to catch up on rest during the daytimes while your baby sleeps. But your baby will only be this sleepy for a few short weeks and he will then increasingly want to be awake, playing and having social time with you and others. He won't know the difference between day and night, and unless you gently guide him into a routine, you could end up with him wide awake and wanting to play games at 4am. So, yes, I do stress the importance of waking the baby every 2–3 hours during the first week to ensure that the breasts are stimulated enough to increase the mother's milk production. Waking the baby three-hourly throughout the day will ensure that the baby will more than likely only wake once in the night between 12pm and 6am. A mother who is well rested and relaxed will be much more likely to produce a more abundant milk supply than a mother who is tired and stressed. In the long term you will both benefit from establishing this pattern.

**Q Several friends and relations have said that it is cruel to wake a sleeping baby and that he will wake up when he is ready to feed. I am a very organised person and feel that following a routine would be best for both my baby and me, but I am frightened that I could do some sort of psychological or physical damage to my baby by waking him.**

**A** It is obvious that the people who say it is cruel to wake a sleeping baby to feed him have never had to care for very premature or sick babies as I have. Waking these babies on a regular basis so they fed little and often was the only way to ensure their survival. Over the years, watching these babies grow up into young children, I have never seen any of them showing any psychological or physical damage. I am convinced that there is a bigger risk of such damage to both baby and mother if a situation arises where a baby is up and demanding to be fed every hour in the night. In the early days I advise feeding a baby little and often to establish breast-feeding. Sometimes this will involve waking him but I advise that, should a young baby demand feeding before three hours, then he must, of course, be fed. A pattern will quickly be established for both you and your baby from which you will both benefit.

**Q The current advice is that parents should have their baby sleep in their room with them for the first six months, but I have heard that you say the baby should be put in his own room from birth. I am concerned that my baby may feel alone and lonely shut away in a dark room by himself for hours at a time.**

A On page 2, I mention that the majority of parents I have worked with have their baby sleep with them in their room at night. Getting your baby settled into his own room sooner rather than later can help you avoid disrupting and unsettling him at some stage down the line when he is used to being in your room. We have all heard tales of parents struggling to get a two-year-old out of their bed. While you and your partner might not mind sharing a room or bed with your baby, you must ask yourself whether you are doing so for your own sake or your baby's. You can make the nursery a peaceful haven for him by using it for nappy changing and naps. Once a bedtime routine is in place, your baby will feel calm and happy as soon as he is taken there. You can always settle him in his cot in his room at 7pm, feed him there again at 10pm and transfer him to your room for the middle-of-the-night feed. I advise new mothers to put their baby down for a nap in a dark, quiet room away from the hustle and bustle. This is for their baby's benefit. While some babies will sleep happily in the midst of a busy household, some may not. How well would we, as adults, sleep in a chair in the middle of a noisy room? Babies will become stressed and exhausted through lack of good, quality sleep. You will also establish a stronger difference between wake time and sleep time when, after a peaceful sleep, you bring him downstairs into the activity of your home for some play time.

**Q Is it true that you say that babies should not be cuddled? I keep reading that babies need lots of physical affection and attention in order for them to feel secure.**

**A** I have always stressed the importance of physical contact and affection with your baby. However, I do say that parents should make sure that the cuddling and affection they give is to satisfy their baby's emotional needs before their own. And, crucially, there is a difference between cuddling your baby and cuddling him to sleep. If he gets used to the latter, it will create a dependence that you will have to break at some point – and it is much easier to get him used to settling himself to sleep at three weeks of age than three months or three years.

**Q While I would like a routine when my baby is born, I do not want to leave him to cry for long spells.**

**A** I would never advise that young babies should be left to cry for lengthy periods of time to get themselves to sleep. I do stress that some babies will fight sleep and they should be allowed 5–10 minutes' 'crying-down' period. They should *never* be left for any longer than this before they are checked again. I also stress that a baby should never be left crying for even 2–3 minutes if there is any doubt that he could be hungry or need winding.

'Crying to sleep' is actually a method that I recommend to use with older babies who have reached six months or a year and are waking several times a night because they have learned the wrong sleep associations, brought on by demand feeding or being rocked or cuddled to sleep. In these instances I recommend a form of sleep training that has been used by childcare experts, paediatricians and health visitors for many years.

In my book, *The Complete Sleep Guide for Contented Babies and Toddlers*, I stress that any form of sleep training is always a last resort to get an older baby to sleep during the night and should only ever be used once parents are absolutely sure that the baby is not waking up because he is hungry. I also advise that before commencing sleep training you should take your baby to see the GP to check there are no medical problems.

The whole aim of the CLB routines is to ensure from the very beginning that the baby's needs are being met so that he does not need to cry for any length of time. The guidelines I give are also to help mothers understand the different reasons why a baby may cry. If a baby is in a routine from a very early age the mother will quickly learn to understand and hence anticipate his needs. I have found that this results in the baby crying very seldom – around 5–10 minutes a day in my experience.

**Q I have read that on your routines a baby should not be fed in the middle of the night once it reaches 12 weeks. Surely all babies are different and a baby should not be forced to go without food if he is really hungry?**

A Some babies, particularly breast-fed babies, may need to be fed once in the middle of the night until they are five or six months old. The majority of babies I have cared for personally would go to sleep during the night (i.e. from the last feed at 11pm to 6–7am) somewhere between eight and 12 weeks. The huge feedback that I receive from readers would indicate that this does seem to be the average age at which babies forming routines would sleep for a longer spell. Each baby, of course, is an individual, but if your baby does not sleep through the night until he is seven months old, neither you nor I nor your baby has 'failed'. My routines are there to help you begin to structure your days and nights, and perseverance will pay off when your baby is ready.

How quickly a baby sleeps through the night is very much determined by his weight and the amount of milk he is capable of drinking at each feed during the day. Some babies who are only capable of drinking small amounts at each feed would obviously need a feed in the night for longer than a baby who is capable of drinking a larger amount at each feed during the day. The aim of the CLB routines is not to push the baby through the night as quickly as possible or to deny the baby a feed in the night if he genuinely needs it. It is to ensure that the baby receives most of his nutritional needs during the day so that when he is physically and mentally ready to go through the night he will automatically do so. The feedback I have had, along with my many years of experience caring for babies, confirms this approach works.

**Q I read a message from a mother in an Internet parenting chatroom that she is very lonely and depressed following your routines as it leaves her no time to get out and meet other mothers.**

**A** I have always said that putting a young baby into a routine can be very demanding on the parents, particularly in the early weeks. However, by the time a baby is 2–3 months of age, a pattern has usually emerged where the baby can stay awake for longer periods during the day and sleep for longer periods at night. In my experience of working with hundreds of mothers, their social outings were certainly restricted for the first 2–3 weeks but after that I cannot recall many mothers who did not manage to meet their friends most afternoons between 2pm and 5pm or for coffee in the mornings. Once you and your baby have got the hang of the routines you can adapt them to suit you all better. The mothers I have worked with have all felt that it is worth putting in the hard work at the beginning because the result is a contented baby who sleeps well at night and enjoys his social times during the day. A mother who has had a good night's sleep will be able to enjoy her days more, too!

I always advise mothers, in the early days, to try and ensure that at least every second day they arrange for a friend or relative to come and visit them so that they do not feel lonely or abandoned. I also stress the importance of a walk every day with the baby to get some fresh air. You can do this with friends – and chatting in the park is also a great way to meet other mums.

**Q In your routines you tell mothers when to eat and drink. This strictness puts me off.**

A You can eat and drink whenever you like! In the early days mothers are often exhausted and put their own needs – even the basics like eating and drinking – at the bottom of their list of priorities. Struggling with a newborn on your own can mean that you find yourself at teatime having only had a piece of toast and half a cup of tea. As a nursing mum, you need to eat plenty of food regularly and to drink plenty of water in order to produce enough milk for your baby and to keep up your own energy levels. I know that many people using my routines refer to the book several times a day so the hours suggested for breakfast, lunch and for drinking lots of water are a reminder not to neglect yourself – and they fit in with what your baby is doing, helping make it easier for you to care for yourself, too.

**Q Why are your routines so rigid? Surely half an hour here or there won't make much difference?**

A *The New Contented Little Baby Book* contains over 10 different routines taking you from week one of your baby's life, right up to the end of his first year. They have been carefully compiled to allow for the fact that your baby will be growing and changing. As he goes through his first three months, he will gradually need less and less daytime sleep as he will be enjoying being awake and playing with you. He needs stimulation and fun during the day. He will need weaning at some point (current guidelines recommend exclusive breast-feeding for six months). His sleeping and feeding needs are constantly changing throughout his first year of life. In my experience, adapting to your baby's changing needs is best done slowly and steadily. My routines are specific in order to help you to make those gradual changes. Once your baby is sleeping for 12 hours every night, you will feel a huge sense of relief and he will be getting the long, deep sleep that he needs for healthy growth and development.

My routines are designed around babies' natural rhythms and they work. You do not have to stick rigidly to them, but half an hour can have a knock-on effect which disrupts the rest of your day and, possibly, your night. For example, if your day begins nearer 8am than 7am, you will find your baby has a later nap at around midday. If he doesn't wake until after 3pm you will find it difficult to get him to settle at 7pm as he is unlikely to be sleepy by then. If the last feed of the day is nearer 8pm, you could find as a result that he does not want his 10pm feed and will wake up in the night. This is certainly not the end of the world occasionally but, over a period of time and as his nutritional needs change, you could find night waking continues, leaving you exhausted and less able to enjoy your baby.

**Q I have been trying to follow your routines for four weeks but my baby is not remotely near fitting in with them. I feel like a failure and wonder if I should just give up and let her feed and sleep whenever she wants.**

**A** It can be very difficult in the early days, and many parents understandably feel it would be easier on them if they let the baby decide what she wants to do. Bear in mind you are recovering from the birth, and looking after a baby, routine or not, is extremely hard work. My routines make sure the hard work is limited to as short a period as possible. Think how hard it would be if your baby was still waking up in the night at nine months old. I can assure you it is worth persevering.

Don't necessarily expect instant contentment, but the result of sticking with the routines in the first weeks is a more enjoyable babyhood and toddlerhood for you and your child. When your baby does fit in, and she will very soon, I can guarantee you will never regret the effort you put in to follow the routines in the first few weeks. The routines are there to help guide you and your baby into what represents the baby's natural patterns and rhythms. Remember that you are not 'failing' if your baby doesn't fit in; just keep going, taking a day at a time. As every experienced parent and grandparent will be telling you – the first few months go very quickly.

Start each day at 7am and attempt to follow the day's routine, but if it has gone pear-shaped by lunchtime, because your baby is wide awake at naptime and sleepy during the social times I suggest, don't panic. Keep repeating the same pattern of feeds and sleeps every day as best you can and your baby will pick it up very soon. If she is crying for food before I say she should be fed and you have tried distracting her or playing with her then you must, of course, feed her. If you really cannot rouse her from a sleep when it's time to play, then leave her a bit longer and don't give yourself or her a hard time. Get up in the morning and try again without feeling you or your baby are getting it 'wrong'. I applaud mums these days who are probably looking after their babies on their own during the days without the support of grannies or aunties up the road. It's very hard work. You are not alone in going through the experience, however, and you are certainly not a failure – it will get better!

**Q Why are you so strict about avoiding eye contact at the 10.30pm feed? I feel very cruel depriving my baby of cuddles and this close contact.**

**A** Please don't deprive your baby of cuddles! Nowhere do I suggest you should not cuddle your baby. On the contrary, a baby who is being held close to his mother, whether breast-fed or bottle-fed, will enjoy his feed more and be ready to return to a contented sleep after he has been winded and settled down quietly. I suggest avoiding eye contact at 10.30pm and during night feeds to help you show your baby gently that this is not play time. Your cuddles can be very close, but overstimulating him at wind-down time can cause him to become overtired and not settle well. He needs his sleep for his mental and physical development and without it he could become fretful, irritable and inconsolable. I feel it is better for the baby to be played with, sung to, shown interesting toys and books when he is wide awake and able to really enjoy himself. Cuddling must be about your baby's needs and not just your own.

**Q Your routines are so strict. When can I enjoy my baby without worrying about what he should be doing next?**

**A** I sincerely hope that every parent enjoys his or her baby, from the first exciting day they come home from hospital, right through babyhood, toddlerhood and beyond. Every day is filled with opportunities for cuddling, playing, singing, reading, splashing in the bath, tickling toes while nappy changing and chatting to your baby. But it is beyond doubt that a contented baby is best able to appreciate and participate in these activities. My routines are there to support and help you find a structure to your days that will result in a contented baby. They are not for everyone, however, and if you feel stressed by following a routine then stop trying. My routines can help you avoid long-term problems such as: overtiredness due to overstimulation; sleep association where a baby has to be rocked to sleep or driven round the block; or continual night wakings which leave you feeling exhausted each morning. Should any of these problems develop, you could turn to my book later on for help.

Bonding evolves slowly over many weeks, and for many mothers without help or support there can be, along with feelings of joy and love for a new baby, feelings of sheer exhaustion, failure and frustration. Nights of broken sleep do not help and mothers often contact me because they feel guilty and resentful that they are not enjoying their babies. Weeks of sleep-deprivation caused by endless middle-of-the-night feeding is bound to hamper bonding and enjoyment of your baby. My routines are there to help you and your baby, not to cause stress, anxiety or feelings of inadequacy. A positive approach to them will help enormously.

**Q I have a toddler as well as a new baby to care for and I cannot seem to get your routines to work around both of them.**

A This is an important point and I have covered it in my book *The Contented Toddler Years*. Many mothers find that school runs or nursery for older children mean that the nap times I suggest are not workable. If you used my routines with your first child, you will at least find the 7am start and 7pm bedtime already established in your household. Your toddler may still take a lunchtime nap if he is under three and this can combine nicely with the baby's nap. You might even get an overlap of half an hour to yourself! I suggest that you concentrate on sticking to my suggested amounts of daytime sleep. So if you have to adapt your baby's daytime sleep around your toddler's routine, try not to let the baby exceed the recommended amount of daily sleep. Then bedtime will at least be guaranteed and you can have an evening to rest and recover from caring for two young children.

# Milk feeding in the first year 3

Milk feeding is of vital importance during the first year of your baby's life. It not only helps lay the foundation for your baby's future health, but it also plays a huge part in how well your child sleeps. Breast milk is without a doubt the best and most natural way to feed your baby. Obviously I cannot give you advice on breast-feeding from a personal perspective, but I am proud to say that the majority of the mothers with whom I have worked managed successfully to breast-feed their babies until solids were introduced, and many even longer than that. Of course, a few of my mothers only managed a few weeks, and others, for personal reasons, chose not to breast-feed at all. I hope that the advice in this book will help you successfully establish breast-feeding for your baby, and even if it does not appeal to you, that you will at least give it a try. Many mothers I have helped who hated breast-feeding their first baby because of the exhaustion of demand feeding, found breast-feeding a complete pleasure when following my CLB routines. If, for some reason, you have already given up or have chosen not to breast-feed, I still offer lots of advice on how to get bottle-feeding right.

The whole aim of my book, and the advice within, is to help and support parents, and in particular mothers, who I know feel a huge amount of pressure these days about giving their baby the best start in life. Of course, breast milk is best, but the reality is that if formula were not a good substitute it would have been banned by the health authorities years ago. So if you have already given up breast-feeding or made a personal informed choice not to, please do not be made to feel guilty by the opinions of others who disapprove. Ignore any nasty comments that you will not bond so closely with your baby because you are not breast-feeding. Speaking from personal experience my own mother only managed to breast-feed me for about 10 days, and no mother and daughter could have been closer than we were. Equally, I have friends who were breast-fed for nearly two years and cannot stand the sight of their mothers!

However, I must stress that, contrary to advice from well-meaning grandmas or aunties, bottle-feeding does not necessarily guarantee you a more contented baby, or make it easier to put him into a routine. Whether your baby is breast-fed or bottle-fed, it will still take time and perseverance to establish a routine, so please do not choose or change your baby's feeding to formula, thinking that you will have a more contented baby. A bottle-fed baby will need as much guidance and help into a routine as a breast-fed one, the only difference being that all the responsibility normally lies with the mother who is breast-feeding. For mothers who wish to breast-feed, the CLB routines will allow you to breast-feed successfully and have a routine, with the bonus of Daddy being able to give your baby a bottle of expressed milk.

## Why breast-feeding goes wrong

The first thing that became obvious to me very early on when working with new mothers, is that while breast-feeding may be the most natural way to feed a newborn baby, for some mothers it does not come easily. Immediately after the birth, midwives encourage mothers to put their baby straight to the breast, and guide them through the techniques of positioning and latching the baby on. For some mothers their baby will latch on to the breast easily, feed well and then drop off to sleep easily until the next feed. For others the baby will fuss and fret, fight the breast or take several sucks before falling asleep. These problems are all very common in the early days.

Mothers are now discharged from hospital within 48 hours of giving birth, and many are sent home without having grasped the basic latching-on techniques that are essential if breast-feeding is to be a success.

When I worked as a maternity nurse I would often arrive at a family's home to find a mother with nipples that were so cracked and bleeding that she would be in tears every time she put the baby to her breast. In situations like this, breast-feeding and bonding get off to a very bad start for both mother and baby. The mother is in a lot of physical pain and also suffers mental agony, thinking she is not a good enough mother because her baby is not latching on properly. The baby gets stressed and cries a lot through hunger, because he is not feeding well enough. All of these problems, and many others associated with breast-feeding, could be avoided if more attention and help were given to the mother in the early days.

I am alarmed by some of the advice being given to new mothers in this country today regarding feeding their newborns. They are told within hours of giving birth that they should use their natural instinct and that their baby will let them know what he needs. I have been fortunate enough to have worked with many families in the Far East and Middle East, where they sometimes seem to know more about what really matters in the early days after the birth, i.e. that both mother and baby need as much help and guidance as possible. The attitude of families from these countries is often totally different from the one we adopt in this country. The mother and baby spend the early days getting as much rest and sleep as possible, and mothers eat a special diet to ensure that they are eating enough of the right foods to help produce a good milk supply. Babies are not just thrust upon their mothers' breasts then left, because 'mother and baby will both do what comes naturally'. Whether it was from a professional outside source, or members of the extended family, the mothers with whom I worked usually had someone to help them with the latching on and feeding position in the early days.

I believe passionately that the way to ensuring more mothers breast-feed successfully is to give them help in the early days. While breast-feeding does come naturally to many mothers, it does not come naturally to all, and we need to take this into account when we give advice.

How milk is produced and the composition of breast milk will also help you understand how the CLB feeding routines can and will work with breast-feeding, provided that you follow the advice on adjusting the routines to meet increased demand during growth spurts, or at times when your baby has not taken a full feed. The following brief summary gives an overview of how breast milk is produced. For more in-depth information I would recommend that you read *What to Expect When You're Breast-Feeding . . . And What If You Can't?* by Clare Byam-Cook.

## Milk production

### Milk let-down reflex

The hormones produced during your pregnancy help prepare your breasts for the production of milk. Once your baby is born and put to the breast to suck, a hormone called oxytocin is released from the pituitary gland at the base of your brain, which sends a 'let-down' signal to the breast. The muscles supporting the milk glands contract and the milk is pushed down the 15 or 20 milk ducts as the baby sucks. Many women feel a slight tingling in their breasts, and their womb contracting when their milk lets down. These feelings normally disappear within a week or two. You may also experience a let-down when you hear your baby cry, or if you think about him when you are apart. If you get tense or are very stressed, oxytocin is not released, making it difficult for your milk to let down. Therefore, it is essential for successful breast-feeding that you feel calm and relaxed. This can be helped by preparing everything needed for a feed in advance. Make sure you are sitting comfortably with your back straight, and the baby well supported. Take time to position him on to the breast correctly. Pain caused by incorrect positioning also affects oxytocin being released, which in turn affects the let-down reflex.

## Milk composition

The first milk your breasts will produce is called colostrum. It is higher in protein and vitamins and lower in carbohydrate and fat than the mature milk that comes in between the third and fifth day. Colostrum also contains some of your antibodies, which will help your baby resist any infections you have had. Compared to the mature milk that soon follows, colostrum is much thicker and looks more yellow. By the second to third day, the breasts are producing a mixture of colostrum and mature milk. Then, somewhere between the third and fifth day, the breasts become engorged, and they will feel very hard, tender and often painful to the touch. This is a sign that the mature milk is fully in. The pain is caused not only by the milk coming in, but also by the enlargement of the milk glands in the breasts and the increased blood supply to the breasts. When the milk comes in, it is essential to feed your baby little and often. Not only will it help stimulate a good milk supply, but it will also help relieve the pain of engorgement. During this time it may be difficult for your baby to latch on to the breast and it may be necessary to express a little milk before feeding. This can be done by placing warm, wet flannels on the breasts and gently expressing a little milk by hand. Many mothers also find some relief by placing the leaves of a chilled cabbage inside their bras between feeds.

Mature milk looks very different from colostrum. It is thinner and looks slightly blue in colour, and its composition also changes during the feed. At the beginning of the feed, your baby gets the fore milk, which is high in volume and low in fat. As the feed progresses, your baby's sucking will slow down and he will pause for longer between sucks. This is a sign that he is reaching the hind milk. Although he only gets a small amount of hind milk, it is very important that he is left on the breast long enough to reach it. It is this hind milk that will help your baby go longer between feeds. If you transfer him to the second breast before he has totally emptied the first breast, he will be more likely to get two lots of fore milk. This will have a knock-on effect and leave him feeling hungry again in a couple of hours. Another feed of fore milk will quickly lead to your baby becoming very 'colicky'. While some babies do not get enough to eat from only one breast and need to be put on the second breast, always check that he has completely emptied the first breast before transferring him (see page 52).

I find that at the end of the first week, by making sure babies are given at least 25 minutes on the first breast, and offered the second breast for 5–15 minutes, I can be sure that they are getting the right balance of fore milk and hind milk. It also ensures that they are content to go between 3–4 hours before demanding their next feed. If your baby is feeding from both breasts at each feed, always remember to start the next feed on the breast you last fed from, so that you can be certain each breast is totally emptied every second feed.

In order to encourage a quick and easy let-down, and to ensure that your baby gets the right balance of fore milk and hind milk, the following guidelines should be followed:

- Make sure that you rest as much as possible between feeds, and that you do not go too long between meals. Also, eat small, healthy snacks between meals.
- Prepare in advance everything needed for the feed: a comfortable chair with arms and a straight back, and perhaps a footstool. Cushions to support both you and the baby, a drink of water and some soothing music will all help towards a relaxing, enjoyable feed for both of you.
- It is essential that you take your time to position the baby on the breast correctly; poor positioning leads to painful and often cracked, bleeding nipples. This, in turn, can affect your let-down and result in a poor feed.
- Always make sure your baby has completely emptied the first

breast before putting him on the second. It is the small amount of high-fat hind milk at the end of a feed that will help your baby go longer between feeds.
- Not all babies need the second breast in the early days. If your baby has totally emptied the first breast, burp him and change his nappy, then offer him the second breast. If he needs more he will take it. If not, start him off on that breast at the next feed.
- If your baby does feed from the second breast, you should still start on that breast at the next feed.
- Once the milk is in and you have built up the time your baby feeds from the breast, it is important that he is on the breast long enough to completely empty it and reach the hind milk. Some babies need up to 30 minutes to completely empty the breast. By gently squeezing your nipple between your thumb and forefinger, you will be able to check if there is any milk still in the breast.
- Never, ever allow your baby to suck on an empty breast; this will only lead to very painful nipples.

## My methods for successful breast-feeding

The key to successful breast-feeding is getting off to the right start, and, as you will have already read, 'little and often' after the birth is essential to helping establish a good milk supply. But putting the baby to the breast little and often will not guarantee you a good milk supply if your baby is not positioned on the breast properly. While in the hospital you will be guided by your midwife and the nurses on how to latch your baby on to the breast. But as you will more than likely leave the hospital within 48 hours of giving birth, I would strongly advise that you get help from an experienced breast-feeding counsellor. There are several organisations which will arrange for someone to visit you in your home and spend time with you while you are feeding your baby to ensure that you are getting the positioning on the breast right. They will, if necessary, make several visits to you to help overcome any problems that you may encounter in the early days.

I would also highly recommend an excellent DVD by one of the leading breast-feeding counsellors in the country. Clare Byam-Cook, author of *What to Expect When You're Breast-feeding . . . And What If You Can't?*, shows how to get to grips with breast-feeding in her DVD.

I advise all my mothers to start on day one by offering five minutes each side every three hours, increasing the time by a few minutes each day until the milk comes in. The three hours is calculated from the beginning of one feed to the beginning of the next feed. Somewhere between the third and fifth day, your milk will be in, and you should have increased the baby's sucking time on the breast to 15–20 minutes. Many babies will now be getting enough milk from the first breast, and be content to go three hours before needing a feed again.

However, if you find your baby is demanding food long before three hours have passed, he should of course be fed, and also offered both breasts at each feed, if he still remains unsettled. Once your milk is in, it is important that you make sure he has emptied the first breast totally before putting him to the second breast. In my experience mothers who change breasts too soon end up feeding their baby too much fore milk, which I believe is one of the main causes of babies never seeming satisfied and suffering from colic. It may take a sleepy baby 20–25 minutes to reach the very important hind milk (which is at least three times fattier than the fore milk) and to empty the breast. Other babies may reach the hind milk much more quickly. Be guided by your baby as to how long he needs to get a good feed. If your baby feeds well, within the times I suggest, is happy and content between feeds and you are getting lots of wet nappies, he is obviously getting enough milk in the time he is on the breast.

*Positioning the baby at the breast*

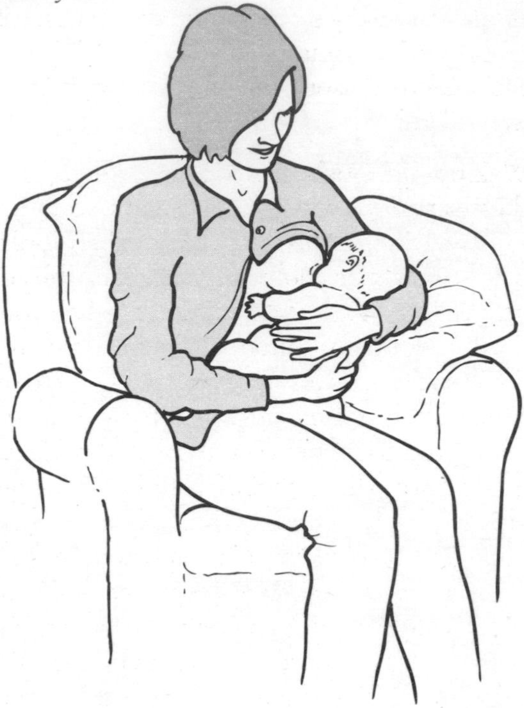

During the first few days, between 6am and midnight, wake your baby every three hours for short feeds. This will ensure that the feeding gets off to the best possible start in time for when the milk comes in. Feeding your baby three-hourly will help build up your milk supply much faster, and if he is fed enough during the day, your baby will be much more likely to go to sleep for longer periods between feeds in the night. It also avoids the mother becoming too exhausted, which, as I've said, is another major factor in breast-feeding going wrong. As with anything in life, success only comes from building a good foundation. All my mothers who establish three-hourly feeds in the hospital find that by the end of the first week a pattern has emerged. Then, very quickly, they can adapt their baby's feeding pattern to my first routine.

The first breast-feeding routine (on page 114) not only helps you establish a good milk supply, but will also enable you to learn all your baby's many different needs: hunger, tiredness, boredom and overstimulation.

The main reasons my breast-feeding methods are so successful are:

- Waking your baby three-hourly in the first few days for shorter periods will gradually allow your nipples to get used to his sucking. This helps avoid the nipples becoming too painful or, even worse, cracked and bleeding. It will also help ease the pain of engorgement when your milk comes in.
- Feeding little and often will help avoid the baby spending hours sucking on an empty breast trying to satisfy his hunger, which often occurs when is a baby is allowed to go longer than three hours between feeds in the first week.
- A newborn baby's tummy is tiny and his needs can only be satisfied by feeding little and often. If you feed your baby three-hourly between 6am and midnight, the 'feeding all night syndrome' should never occur. Even if a very small baby is capable of going one longer spell in between feeds, following my advice ensures that this will happen to all babies at night and not during the day.
- Successful breast-feeding can only be achieved if a mother feels relaxed and comfortable. This is impossible if, having just given birth, you become exhausted from being awake and feeding all night.
- Newborn babies do not know the difference between day and night. Your baby will learn the difference much sooner if you differentiate between daytime feeding and night-time feeding and do not allow him to sleep for long spells between feeds from 7am to 7pm.

## Expressing

I believe that expressing milk in the early days plays a huge part in determining how successful a mother will be in breast-feeding while following a routine. I am convinced that one of the main reasons the majority of my mothers are so successful at breast-feeding is because I encourage the use of an electric expressing machine in the very early days.

The simple reason for this is that breast milk is produced on a supply and demand basis. During the very early days, most babies will empty the first breast and some may take a small amount from the second breast. Very few will empty both breasts at this stage. By the end of the second week, the milk production balances out and most mothers are producing exactly the amount their baby is demanding. Some time during the third and fourth week, the baby goes through a growth spurt and demands more milk. This is where a problem often sets in if you are attempting to put your baby into a routine and have followed the current advice of not expressing before six weeks.

In order to meet the increased demand for more food, you would more than likely have to go back to feeding two- or three-hourly and often twice in the night. This feeding pattern is repeated each time the baby goes through a growth spurt and often results in the baby being continually fed just prior to sleep time. This can create the problem of the wrong sleep association, making it even more difficult to get the baby back into the routine.

Mothers who express the extra milk they produce in the very early days will always be producing more than their baby needs. When their baby goes through a growth spurt, the routine stays intact, because simply expressing less milk at the early-morning feeds can immediately satisfy any increased appetite.

Expressing from the very early days can also help avoid the problem of a low milk supply. However, if your baby is over one month and you already have the problem of a low milk supply, by following my plan for increasing your milk supply (page 213), you should see a big improvement within six days. For babies under one month, following the expressing times laid out in the routines should be enough to increase your supply.

If you decide some time between one and four weeks to introduce a bottle (see page 101) of either expressed milk or formula at the 10.30pm feed, you will be able to hand over feeding responsibility to someone else. This means that you will be able to get to bed early if you are feeling exhausted from night feeding. I advise in my routines that you express some milk at this time *or* that you feed the baby. If the baby takes a bottle, then you can express between 9.30–10pm and then go to bed. Expressing milk at this time is important to keep the supply going and ensure you have plenty for the middle-of-the-night feed.

If you have previously experienced difficulties with expressing, do not be disheartened. Expressing at the time suggested in my routines or the plan in the chapter on common problems, along with the following guidelines, should help make it easier:

- The best time to express is in the morning as the breasts are usually fuller. Expressing will also be easier if done at the beginning of a feed. Express one breast just prior to feeding your baby, or feed your baby from one breast, then express from the second breast before offering him the remainder of his feed. Some mothers actually find that expressing is easier when done while they are feeding the baby on the other breast. It is also important to note that expressing at the beginning of a feed allows slightly longer for that breast to make more milk for the next feed.

  In my routines I suggest that the mother expresses at 6.45am; however, if you are producing a lot of milk and can't face the early morning slot, you could move the expressing of the second breast to around 7.30am after the baby has fed from the first breast. A mother who is concerned about her milk supply or who is following the plan for increasing the milk (on page 213) should try to stick to the recommended times.
- In the early days, you will need to allow at least 15 minutes to express 60–90ml (2–3oz) at the morning feeds, and up to

30 minutes at the evening expressing times. Try to keep expressing times quiet and relaxed. The more you practise, the easier it will become. I usually find that, by the end of the first month, the majority of my mothers can easily express 60–90ml (2–3oz) within 10 minutes at the 10pm expressing when using a double pumping system.
- An electrical, heavy-duty pumping machine, the type used in hospitals, is by far the best way to express milk in the early days. The suction of these machines is designed to simulate a baby's sucking rhythm, encouraging the milk flow. If you are expressing both breasts at 10pm, it is also worthwhile investing in an attachment that enables both breasts to be expressed at once, therefore reducing the time spent expressing.
- Sometimes, the let-down is slower in the evening when the breasts are producing less milk; a relaxing warm bath or shower will often help encourage the milk to flow more easily. Also, gently massaging the breasts before and during expressing will help.
- Some mothers find that it is helpful to have a picture of their baby close by for them to look at, while others find it better to watch a favourite television programme, or to chat to their partners or husbands. Experiment with different approaches to see which one works best for you.

As you proceed through the routines I advise which expressing times to drop. You cut back on expressing as your milk supply becomes firmly established. By three months you will only be expressing at the 10pm feed and, some time between four and six months, you can cut this final expressing out. Once your milk supply is reliably established to suit your baby you can be flexible with the 10pm expressing. If you don't do it some nights, it won't be a problem. I advise continuing to express into the fourth and fifth month so you have extra milk to give your baby as he shows signs of needing weaning. If you decide to wean before six months (after advice from a health professional) you can stop expressing straight away.

# Breast-feeding and returning to work

If you are planning to return to work and would like to continue to breast-feed, it is important that you try to make sure that you have established a good milk supply, especially if you want your baby to have expressed breast milk during the day. A three-month-old baby will need two feeds of approximately 210–240ml (7–8oz) each of expressed milk if you are out between 9am and 5pm. As your baby will most likely be emptying both breasts at the 7am and 6pm feeds, you will need to express most of the milk for the feeds to be given in your absence during the working day or between 9pm and 10pm in the evening.

You should fit in two expressing sessions at around 10am and 2.30pm. If you express any later than this, it is possible that your breasts will not produce enough for the 6pm feed, especially if you are in a hurry to get home.

The following guidelines give suggestions on how to incorporate working and breast-feeding:

- The longer you can spend at home establishing a milk supply, the easier it will be to maintain it once you return to work. Most breast-feeding experts advise a period of 16 weeks.
- Expressing from the beginning of the second week at the times suggested will enable you to build up a good stock of breast milk in the freezer.
- Introducing a bottle of expressed milk at the 10pm feed by the second week will ensure that there will not be a problem of your baby not taking the bottle when you return to work.
- Check with your employer well in advance of returning to work that there will be a quiet place available where you will be able to express. Also check that they are happy for you to store the expressed milk in the refrigerator.
- Once you have established a good expressing routine using the heavy-duty expressing pump, you should begin

practising with a battery-operated one. With a single expressing pump you may find that switching from side to side throughout the expressing will help the milk to flow more easily. It may also be worthwhile considering a mini-electric pump that will enable you to express both breasts at once.

- Make sure that the nursery, or your nanny or child-minder, is familiar with the storage and handling of breast milk, and how to defrost it.
- Establish the combined feeding routine that you will be using for your baby at least two weeks in advance of your return to work. This will allow you plenty of time to sort out any difficulties that may occur.
- Once you return to work, it is essential that you pay particular attention to your diet and that you rest well in the evening. It would be advisable to continue expressing at 10pm to ensure that you maintain a good milk supply. Also, make sure that you keep a good supply of breast pads at work, and a spare shirt or top!

## Weaning your baby from the breast to the bottle

However long you have breast-fed, it is important to plan the transition from breast-feeding to bottle-feeding properly. When deciding for how long you intend to breast-feed your baby, you should take into consideration that once you have established a good milk supply, you must allow approximately a week to drop each feed. For example, it can take six weeks to establish a good milk supply, and if you decide to give up breast-feeding, you should allow, at the very least, a further five weeks to drop all breast-feeds and establish bottle-feeding. This information is very important for mothers who are planning to go back to work. If you give up breast-feeding before you have established a good milk supply, you should still allow enough time for your baby to get used to feeding from the bottle. Some babies can get very upset if they suddenly lose the pleasure and comfort they get from breast-feeding.

For a mother who has breast-fed for less than a month, I generally advise a period of 3–4 days in between dropping feeds. For a mother who has been breast-feeding longer than a month, it is best to allow 5–7 days in between dropping feeds. Assuming that the baby is already on a bottle-feed at 10.30pm, the next breast-feed to drop should be at 11am. The best way to do this is gradually to reduce the length of time the baby feeds from the breast by five minutes each day and top up with formula. Once your baby is taking a full bottle-feed, the breast-feed can be dropped. If you plan the weaning carefully from the breast to formula, your baby will have time to adjust to the bottle and you avoid the risk of developing mastitis. This can happen if the milk ducts become blocked due to engorgement, a common problem among mothers who instantly drop a feed.

I suggest that you continue to express at 10pm throughout the weaning process. The amount of milk expressed will be an indicator of how quickly your milk supply is going down.

Some mothers find that once they are down to two breast-feeds a day, their milk reduces very rapidly. The signs to watch out for are: your baby being irritable and unsettled after a feed; or wanting a feed long before it is normally due. If your baby shows either of these signs, he should be topped up immediately after the breast-feed with 30–60ml (1–2oz) of expressed milk or formula. This will ensure that his sleeping pattern does not go wrong due to hunger.

The chart below is a guideline for which feeds to drop first. Each stage represents the period of time between dropping feeds – either 3–4 days or 5–7 days, depending on how long you have been breast-feeding.

| *Time of feeds* | *7am* | *11am* | *2.30pm* | *6.30pm* | *10pm* |
|---|---|---|---|---|---|
| **Stage one** | Breast | Formula | Breast | Breast | Express* |
| **Stage two** | Breast | Formula | Formula | Breast | Express |
| **Stage three** | Breast | Formula | Formula | Formula | Express |
| **Stage four** | Breast | Formula | Formula | Formula | |
| **Stage five** | Formula | Formula | Formula | Formula | |

* I recommend that mothers should continue to express at the 10.30pm feed (provided the baby is taking his bottle from his father or another helper) until the baby is 3–4 months old. This helps maintain a good milk supply, and can be used as an approximate gauge of how much milk they are producing. I find that a mother will usually produce overnight roughly twice the amount she has expressed. When you reach stage three of the weaning process, the 10pm expressing should be dropped gradually, reducing the expressing time by three minutes each night. Once you are only expressing 60ml (2oz) and going comfortably through the night, the expressing can be dropped altogether. When the last breast-feed has been dropped, care should be taken not to stimulate the breasts. Sitting in a warm bath with the water covering the breasts helps to get rid of any small amount of milk remaining in the breasts without stimulating them to make more.

## Bottle-feeding

If you have decided to bottle-feed, the same routines as for breast-feeding should be followed. The only difference is that you may find your baby is happy to go longer than three hours after the 7am feed, otherwise the timing is exactly the same. In the instances where a feed is being split – i.e. one breast before the bath and one after – the same pattern applies to bottle-feeding. I would normally make up two separate smaller feeds for this time.

### How much and how often?

Health authorities advise that a baby under four months would need 70ml (2½oz) of milk for each pound of his body weight; a baby weighing around 3.2kg (7lb) would need approximately 510ml (17oz) a day. This is only a guideline; hungrier babies may need an extra ounce at some feeds. If your baby is one of these try to ensure that you structure your feeds so he is taking the bigger feeds at the right times, i.e. 7am, 10.30am or 10.30pm. If you allow him to get into the habit of having bigger feeds in the middle of the night, it would eventually have the knock-on effect of him not being so hungry when he wakes in the morning. A vicious circle emerges where he needs to feed in the night because he does not feed enough during the day.

The same guidelines apply as for breast-feeding: aim to get the baby to take most of his daily milk requirements between 7am and 11pm. This way he will only need a small feed in the middle of the night, and will eventually drop it altogether.

The chart below is an example of the feeding pattern of one of my babies during his first month. He weighed 3.2kg (7lb) at birth and, with a weekly gain of 180–240g (6–8oz), reached just over 4kg (9lb) when he was one month old. By structuring the feeding (the bigger feeds at the right times) he was well on the way to dropping his middle-of-the-night feed, and at six weeks he was sleeping through to 6.30am.

| *Times* | *7am* | *10 – 10.30am* | *2– 2.30pm* | *5pm* | *6.15pm* | *10– 11pm* | *2– 3am* | *Total* |
|---|---|---|---|---|---|---|---|---|
| **Week 1** | **90ml** (3oz) | **90ml** (3oz) | **90ml** (3oz) | **60ml** (2oz) | **60ml** (2oz) | **90ml** (3oz) | **90ml** (3oz) | **570ml** (19oz) |
| **Week 2** | **90ml** (3oz) | **120ml** (4oz) | **90ml** (3oz) | **90ml** (3oz) | **60ml** (2oz) | **120ml** (4oz) | **60ml** (2oz) | **630ml** (22oz) |
| **Week 3** | **120ml** (4oz) | **120ml** (4oz) | **90ml** (3oz) | **90ml** (3oz) | **90ml** (3oz) | **120ml** (4oz) | **90ml** (3oz) | **720ml** (24oz) |
| **Week 4** | **150ml** (5oz) | **120ml** (4oz) | **120ml** (4oz) | **90ml** (3oz) | **90ml** (3oz) | **150ml** (5oz) | **60ml** (2oz) | **780ml** (26oz) |

**N.B.** These daily amounts of milk were calculated to suit that particular baby's needs. Remember to adjust the quantities of milk to suit your baby's own needs, but still follow the feeding times shown. During growth spurts make sure that the 7am, 10.30am and 10–11pm feeds are the first to be increased.

## Establishing bottle-feeding

When your baby is born, the hospital may provide you with ready-made formula. You may be given a choice of two different brands; both are approved by the health authorities and there is very little difference in the composition of either milk. The bottles of formula will come with pre-packed sterilised teats, which are used once and then thrown away.

Unless the jars have been stored in the fridge they do not need to be heated; they can be given at room temperature. However, if for some reason you do decide to heat the formula, do so by using either an electric bottle-warmer or by standing it in a jug of boiling water.

Never heat the formula in a microwave, as the heat may not be evenly distributed and you could end up by scalding your baby's mouth. Whichever form of heating you use, always test the temperature before giving the bottle to your baby. This can be done by shaking a few drops on the inside of your wrist; it should feel lukewarm, never hot. Once milk is heated, it should never be reheated, as this very rapidly increases the bacteria levels in the milk, which is one of the main causes of upset tummies in formula-fed babies.

The advice given in hospital for formula-fed babies seems to be much the same as for breast-fed babies: 'Feed on demand whenever the baby wants and however much he wants.' While you do not have the problem of establishing a milk supply as in breast-feeding, many of the other problems are likely to occur. A bottle-fed baby weighing 3.2kg (7lb) or more at birth could go straight on to the 2–4-week routine, for example. A smaller baby might not manage to last quite as long between feeds and need feeding nearer three-hourly.

Ready-made formula is incredibly expensive to use all the time; most parents only use it on outings or in emergencies. Before leaving the hospital, arrange for someone to buy at least two large tins of powdered formula milk of the same brand as the ready-made milk to which your baby has been introduced at the hospital. Make sure it is appropriate for newborns.

Once home, you will get into a routine of making up in advance the feeds needed for the next 24 hours. When making up the formula, choose a quiet time of the day when you are not too tired and follow the instructions on the tin very carefully. Any feeds left over from the previous day should be discarded; likewise, never save unfinished feeds. After a feed has been heated up it should be used within one hour and any remaining after this time should be thrown out and, if necessary, a fresh feed heated up. In the early days it is advisable to have an extra bottle of boiled water in the fridge, ready for emergencies. Water left out of the fridge should be okay provided it is used within a few hours. However, if the weather is hot I would not leave it out for long.

## Hygiene and sterilisation

The utmost attention must be paid to hygiene: the sterilising of all your baby's feeding equipment and the preparation and storing of his formula milk.

The area where you sterilise and prepare your baby's formula should be kept spotlessly clean. Every morning the work-top should be thoroughly washed down with hot soapy water, the cloth used should then be rinsed well under hot running water and the surface wiped again to remove any traces of soap. This should be followed by a final wipe-down using kitchen roll and antiseptic spray.

The guidelines below, if applied to the letter, will reduce the risk of germs, which are so often the cause of tummy upsets in very young babies:

- Surfaces should be washed down thoroughly every day, as described above.
- After each feed the bottle and teat should be rinsed out thoroughly using cold water, and put aside in a bowl ready for washing and sterilising.
- Get into the habit of sterilising and preparing feeds at the same time every day. Choose a time when you are not too tired and are able to concentrate properly. Most of my mothers find that 12 noon, when the baby has gone for his long nap, is a good time.
- Hands should always be washed thoroughly with anti-bacterial soap under warm running water, then dried with kitchen roll, not a tea towel, which is a breeding ground for germs.
- A separate kettle can be kept for boiling the baby's water;

this avoids the water accidentally being boiled a second time if someone wants to make a cup of tea.

- Every day empty the kettle and rinse it out. The water from the tap should be allowed to run for a couple of minutes before filling the kettle.
- Boil the water first, so that it has time to cool while you are washing and sterilising the bottles.
- Throw away any feeds in the fridge that are left over from the previous 24 hours.
- Fill the bowl in which the dirty bottles are stored with hot, soapy water. Using a long-handled bottle brush, carefully scrub all the bottles, rims, caps and teats inside and out. Particular attention should be given to the necks and rims. Carefully rinse everything under a hot running tap. Wash and rinse the bowl thoroughly, then place all the equipment in the bowl under the running hot water tap. This is to check that everything is thoroughly rinsed – the water should run clear.
- The steriliser should be rinsed out every day, and the removable parts checked and, if necessary, washed and rinsed. The bottles and teats should then be packed into the steriliser following the manufacturer's instructions.
- When the water in the kettle is cool and the bottles sterilised, carefully follow the instructions on the tin of formula and make up enough feeds for the next 24 hours.

### Giving the feed

Prepare everything in advance: chair, cushions, bib and muslin. As with breast-feeding, it is important that you are sitting comfortably (see page 6), and in the early days I advise all mothers to support the arm in which they are holding the baby with a pillow, which enables you to keep the baby on a slight slope with his back straight. By holding the baby as shown in diagram A (opposite), you will lessen the likelihood of your baby getting air trapped in his tummy, which he might if fed as shown in diagram B.

*Positioning of your baby while bottle-feeding*

Diagram A: Correct

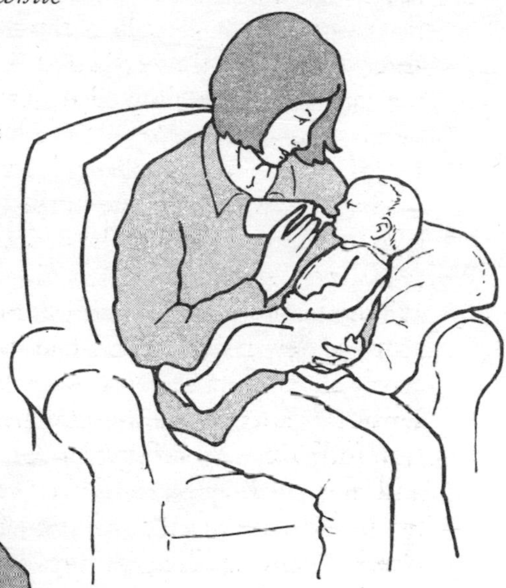

Diagram B: Incorrect

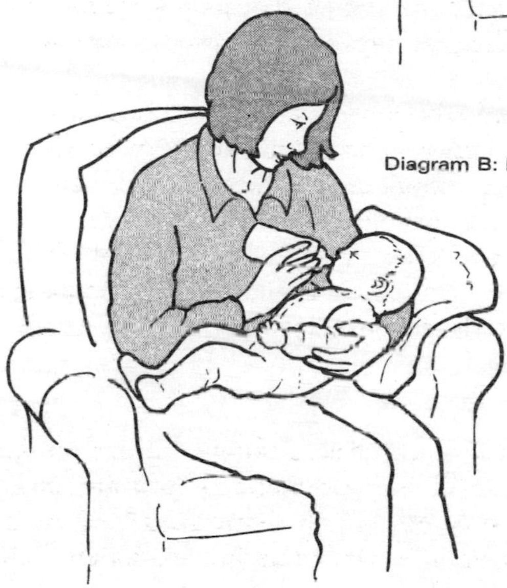

Before starting to feed, loosen and screw the teat back on; it should be very slightly loose. If it is screwed on too tightly it will not allow air into the bottle, and your baby will end up sucking and not getting any milk.

Check also that the milk is not too hot; it should be just slightly warm. If you get your baby used to very warm milk, you will find that, as the feed progresses and the milk gets cool, he will refuse to feed. As it is dangerous to reheat the milk or keep it standing in hot water for any length of time, you could end up having to heat up two bottles for every feed.

Once feeding, make sure that the bottle is kept tilted up far enough to ensure that the teat is always filled with milk, to prevent your baby taking in too much air. Allow your baby to drink as much as he wants before stopping to burp him. If you try to burp him before he is ready he will only get very cross and upset.

Some babies will take most of their feed, burp and then want a break of 10–15 minutes before finishing the remainder of the milk. In the early days, allowing for a break midway, it can take up to 40 minutes to give the bottle. Once your baby is 6–8 weeks old he will most likely finish his feed in about 20 minutes.

If you find your baby is taking a very long time to feed, or keeps falling asleep halfway through a feed, it could be because the hole in the teat is too small. I find that many of my babies have to go straight on to a medium-flow teat as the slow-flow one is too slow.

Occasionally there are babies who will drink a full feed in 10–15 minutes and look for more. These babies are often referred to as 'hungrier babies'; the reality is that these babies are usually 'sucky' babies, not hungrier ones. Because they have such a strong suck they are able to finish the bottle very quickly. Sucking is not only a means of feeding to a baby, but, in the early days, one of their natural pleasures. If your baby is taking the required amount of formula at each feed very quickly and looking for more, it may be worthwhile trying a teat with a smaller hole. Offering him a dummy after feeds may also help satisfy his 'sucking needs'.

It is very easy for bottle-fed babies to gain weight too quickly if they are allowed to have feeds well in excess of the amounts recommended for their weight. While a few ounces a day should not create a problem, a baby who is overeating, and regularly putting on more than 240g (8oz) each week, will eventually become too fat and reach a stage where milk alone is not enough to satisfy his hunger. If this happens before the recommended age for giving solids, it can create a real problem.

For establishing successful bottle-feeding the following guidelines should be observed:

- Before beginning the feed, check that the ring holding the teat and the bottle together is very slightly loose; if it is too tight it will restrict the flow of the milk.
- Check that the milk is the right temperature; it should be lukewarm, not hot.
- To avoid wind problems, which are very common among formula-fed babies, always make sure that you are comfortable and holding your baby correctly before beginning the feed.
- Some very young babies need a break in the middle of the feed. Allow up to 40 minutes for your baby to take a full feed.
- If you find you are having always to wake your baby for the 7am feed, only to find he is not so hungry, then cut back the middle-of-the-night feed by 30ml (1oz).
- During growth spurts, make sure you follow the guidelines in the next section. This will avoid your baby cutting back, or even dropping, the wrong feeds first.

## Formula: overfeeding

Unlike the breast-fed baby, the most common problem in the early days with formula-fed babies is overfeeding. The reason I believe this can happen with some babies is that they take the bottle of formula so quickly that their natural sucking instincts are not satisfied and they end up screaming when the bottle is removed from their mouth. Many mothers interpret this cry as one of hunger and end up giving them another bottle of formula. A pattern of overfeeding can quickly emerge, resulting in the baby gaining huge amounts of weight each week. If this problem is allowed to continue, the baby quickly reaches a stage where milk alone will not satisfy his appetite, yet he is too young to be given solids (under six months).

While it is normal for some babies to need an additional 30ml (1oz) at some feeds, special attention should be given if a baby is taking in excess of 150ml (5oz) every day, and is regularly gaining more than 240g (8oz) each week. When my formula-fed babies show signs of being particularly 'sucky', I have found that offering some cool boiled water between feeds and a dummy afterwards helps to satisfy their sucking needs.

If you are concerned that your baby is overfeeding, it is essential that you discuss the problem with your health visitor or doctor.

## Your questions answered

**Q I have very small breasts and am worried that I may not be able to produce enough milk to satisfy my baby's needs.**

A
- Breast size is totally irrelevant when it comes to producing breast milk. Each breast, regardless of shape or size, has 15–20 ducts, each duct with its own cluster of milk-making cells. Milk is made within these cells and pushed down the ducts when the baby sucks.
- During the early days, make sure your baby is put to the breast frequently. Most babies need a minimum of eight feeds a day to help stimulate the breasts and establish a good milk supply.
- Always make sure that your baby totally empties the first breast before putting him on the second breast. This signals the breast to make more milk and also ensures that your baby gets the important hind milk.

**Q My friend was in agony when her milk came in. Is there anything I can do to help relieve the pain of engorgement?**

A
- Put your baby to the breast often and do not let him go longer than three hours during the day between feeds or 4–5 hours at night.

- A warm bath or warm wet flannels placed on the breasts before a feed will help the milk flow and, if need be, gently expressing a little milk by hand will make it easier for the baby to latch on.
- Damp flannels chilled in the fridge and placed on the breasts after a feed will help constrict the blood vessels and reduce the swelling.
- Take the leaves just under the outer leaves of a cabbage, chill in the fridge and place on your breasts inside your bra between feeds.
- Wear a well-fitting nursing bra that supports your breasts. Make sure that it is not too tight under the arms and does not flatten your nipples.

**Q Many of my friends had to give up breast-feeding because it was so painful.**

A
- The main reason women experience pain in the early days is because the baby is not positioned on the breast correctly. The baby ends up chewing on the end of the nipple, causing much pain for the mother, more often than not resulting in cracked, bleeding nipples and a poor feed for the baby. A pattern soon emerges of the baby needing to feed again very quickly, giving him even more opportunity to damage the nipples.
- Make sure that you always hold your baby with his tummy to your tummy and that his mouth is open wide enough for him to take all of the nipple and as much of the areola as he can manage into his mouth. Apart from ensuring that your baby is well positioned, it is important that you are sitting comfortably. The ideal chair should have a straight back, preferably with arms so that you can position a cushion to support the arm in which you are holding the baby (see page 6). If you do not support your arm, it will be much more difficult to position and support your baby properly. This can cause him to pull on the breast, which will be painful for you.

**Q I have a three-week-old baby and am getting very concerned over the conflicting advice. Some people say give both breasts at each feed, others say one is enough.**

A
- Be guided by your baby. If he feeds from one breast, is content to go 3–4 hours between feeds, and is putting on 180–240g (6–8oz) in weight each week, one breast is obviously enough.
- If he is looking for food after two hours, or is waking up in the night more than once, it would be advisable to offer him the second breast. You may find he only needs the second breast later in the day when your milk supply is at its lowest.
- Whether your baby has one or two breasts at a feed, always check that the first breast is completely empty before putting him on the second. This can be done by gently squeezing the area around the nipple between your thumb and forefinger.

**Q Do I need to avoid certain foods while breast-feeding?**

A
- You should continue with the same varied, healthy diet that you followed throughout your pregnancy. In addition, you should include small healthy snacks between meals to help keep your energy levels up.
- Ensure that you eat at least 180g (6oz) of either poultry, lean meat or fish. Vegetarians should eat the equivalent in beans, pulses and rice etc. I have noticed that on the days when some of my breast-feeding mothers did not eat enough protein, their babies were much more unsettled.
- Some research points to dairy products as the cause of colic in certain babies. If you find your baby develops colic, it may be wise to discuss how to monitor your dairy intake with your health visitor or paediatrician.
- Alcohol, artificial sweeteners and caffeine should be avoided. Remember that caffeine is not only found in coffee, but also in tea, soft drinks and chocolate. I have found all of these things can upset most babies.
- Strawberries, tomatoes, mushrooms, onions and fruit

juice, if taken in large quantities, have left many of my babies very irritable. While I do not suggest cutting out all of these from your diet, I would suggest that you keep a record of any food or drink consumed 12–16 hours prior to your baby showing signs of tummy ache, explosive bowel movements, excessive wind and crying fits.

- While working in the Middle and Far East, I observed that breast-feeding mothers followed a much blander diet than normal, and that highly spiced foods were omitted. Perhaps it would be wise to avoid curries in the early days.
- Although it is advisable to avoid alcohol, especially spirits, while breast-feeding, some experts advise that a small glass of wine or a Guinness can be beneficial to a mother who is finding it hard to unwind in the evening.

**Q My two-week-old baby wakes up yelling for a feed, only to fall asleep after five minutes on the breast. He then demands to be fed two hours later, leaving me absolutely exhausted.**

A
- Always make sure your baby is fully awake before you attempt to feed him. Unwrap him in the cot, take his legs out of his baby-grow and allow the cool air to get to his skin, and give him time to wake up by himself. Then you can start his feed.
- It is very important that sleepy babies are kept cool while feeding. He should not be overdressed and the room should not be too warm. Have a play mat next to you on the floor and the minute he gets sleepy, put him on it. If necessary, remove his baby-grow, as this will encourage him to stretch and kick. Within a few minutes he will probably protest about being put down, so pick him up and give him a few more minutes on the same breast. This procedure often has to be repeated two or three times. Once he has had 20 minutes on the first breast, burp him well and change his nappy. He can then be put back on the first breast if he has not emptied it, or transferred to the second.

- If you are not using formula at the 10.30pm feed, it is also a good idea to express some milk early in the morning and get your partner to do the 10.30pm feed. This way, you will at least manage to get an uninterrupted few hours' sleep for one part of the night.

**Q My son is 16 weeks old. Over the last two weeks he has become increasingly difficult to feed. He dropped the middle-of-the-night feed at around 11 weeks old yet, despite not feeding after 10.30pm, he is fairly disinterested in his 7am feed, taking as little as 60ml (2oz). He then cries on and off until I feed him at 11am. When I feed him earlier than 11am he then does not sleep well at lunchtime, waking up after an hour looking for a feed. When I feed him then, it puts the rest of the feeds out for the afternoon.**

A

- To get your son more interested in his 7am feed try cutting back on his 10.30pm feed. Although he will need a small feed at this time, probably until he is weaned on to solids, try reducing it gradually to 90–120ml (3–4oz) and see if he is more interested at 7am. If this helps him feed better at 7am then continue to reduce the amount he takes then to 90–120ml (3–4oz).
- Until he is feeding better at 7am you will have to feed him earlier than 11am, possibly by 10.15am, but I would suggest that you top him up around 11.15/11.30am to ensure that he has taken enough milk to ensure he sleeps well at his lunchtime nap.
- You may also find that when he goes through a growth spurt he starts to take his morning bottle much more quickly and may even start waking up earlier, looking for a feed. When this happens I would suggest that you go back to giving him more at the 10.30pm feed to ensure he gets through to 7am. You may have to do this for a week or so, and perhaps even continue with a larger feed until he is weaned. However, if he started to get fussy about the morning feed again, you would then have to cut back on the 10.30pm feed once more.

# Understanding your baby's sleep 4

Sleep is probably the most misunderstood and confusing aspect of parenthood. The misconception is that for the first few weeks all the baby will do is feed and sleep. While many do, the fact that there are over 126 sleep clinics in the United Kingdom for babies and children is proof that a great many do not. If your newborn or young baby is one of the latter – tense, fretful and difficult to settle – please take heart, as this need not be a reflection of your baby's future sleep habits.

The majority of babies that I helped care for personally usually started to sleep to 6–7am somewhere between eight and 12 weeks. A few slept through before that age and some still needed to be fed in the night for much longer. As I do not know your baby personally, I cannot give you a specific answer as to when he will sleep through, as many factors will dictate that. For example, if your baby was born prematurely or you did not start following the routines until he was several weeks old, then obviously he may take longer to sleep through the night.

The important thing to remember is that what you are trying to achieve in the early days is a regular sleeping pattern, where your baby settles well in the evening, feeds and settles at 10.30pm, and then only wakes once in the night for a feed and goes back to sleep quickly until 6–7am.

The aim of the routines is to achieve this without causing distress to you or your baby; they are not about pushing your baby through the night at the earliest possible age without feeding him. By following the guidelines I have laid out in this book, and adjusting the routines if need be to suit your baby's own particular needs, he will sleep the longest spell at night as soon as he is physically and mentally capable of doing so.

The key to achieving this is to be patient, consistent and allow time for my routines to become established. Once they are, you can avoid the agony of months of sleepless nights that so many parents go through. It has worked for hundreds of thousands of babies and their parents, so it can work for you!

If you want your baby to sleep through the night from an early age and ensure a long-term healthy sleep pattern, the golden rules are **to establish the right associations, and to structure your baby's feeds from the day you arrive home from the hospital**. The advice given in many of the baby books, and by some hospital staff, is that newborn babies should feed on demand for as often and for as long as they need. You will be told to accept that your baby's erratic sleeping and feeding patterns are normal and that things will improve by three months of age. Since the publication of my first book in 1999 I have received countless phone calls, emails and letters from distraught mothers whose infants, aged anywhere between three months and three years, have serious sleep and feeding problems. This continually disproves the theory that babies will put themselves into a routine by three months. Even if a baby does do this, it is unlikely to be a routine that fits in with the rest of the family.

While some experts agree that some babies are capable of sleeping through the night by three months, they do not stress the importance of guiding the baby towards this goal. The innocent and weary mother believes in and hopes for a miraculous improvement at three months, but this is unlikely to happen if her baby has not learned the difference between day and night, naps and the long sleep, and if the parent has not learned how to structure feeds, which needs to be established from day one. Ensuring that your baby feeds little and often during the day is essential if you want to avoid his waking up genuinely hungry every couple of hours during the night.

When I ran my consultancy service for new parents I would, on a daily basis, receive desperate calls from the maternity wards. The cry for help was nearly always the same. The baby is feeding for up to an hour at a time, usually two-hourly from 6pm until 5am. The mother is often exhausted and starting to suffer from cracked nipples.

When I ask what the baby is like during the day the usual reply is: 'He's ever so good during the day; he will feed then go four hours or longer.'

It continues to baffle me that such contradictory advice is still being given to new parents. They are told that it is normal for a newborn baby to need to feed as much as 8–12 times a day, but they should then allow the baby to sleep hours between daytime feeds. It is hardly surprising that a baby who has had only four or even fewer feeds between 6am and 6pm is going to wake up many times in the night to satisfy his daily needs. This is one of the main reasons that I am opposed to the advice that babies should be demand fed. It does not take into account that many babies do not demand to be fed in the early days.

## Sleep and demand feeding

The phrase 'demand feeding' is used time and time again, misleading a mother into believing that any sort of routine in the early days could deny her baby nutritionally and, according to some experts, emotionally. While I would totally agree that the old-fashioned four-hourly routine of feeding, whether breast or bottle, is not natural to newborn babies, I feel the term 'feeding on demand' is used too loosely.

The pattern for sleepless nights is unfortunately often set before mother and baby leave the hospital. Because the baby has been allowed to sleep for long spells between feeds during the day, he genuinely needs to feed on and off all evening and every couple of hours in the night. A vicious circle soon emerges where the baby is sleeping for most of the day because he has been awake most of the night. This type of sleeping and feeding pattern is encouraged by many experts as they believe that the baby should take the lead where feeding is concerned. Hence the terms 'baby-led feeding' or 'demand feeding'. Some experts even go as far as to say that it is 'damaging' to wake a sleeping baby, and take a very hostile view of my advice to do so. It was my experience of working with many sets of twins and premature babies that helped me to realise this was complete nonsense. I observed that when I went to care for these babies, the hospital staff had already implemented a feeding routine. Because the lives of these tiny, sleepy babies depended on being fed little and often, they would not have dared take the risk of allowing them to go long spells between feeds. This experience went a long way in helping me develop the CLB routines. Contrary to what some people try to imply, the routines are not about denying the baby food, but about ensuring that they are fed enough. As I have already mentioned, I have had personal experience of caring for babies who nearly lost their lives due to dehydration, because they were not demanding to be fed enough. This further convinced me that demand-feeding puts a baby at much more risk than if the baby is woken at regular intervals and offered a feed.

Because breast milk is produced on a supply and demand basis – i.e the breasts make the amount of milk that the baby demands – within a few weeks the demand-fed baby often starts to demand to be fed two-hourly not only at night but during the day as well. This is because the feeding pattern of the previous 2–3 weeks has affected the supply of breast milk. Because the baby is feeding so often it is inevitable that, more often than not, the baby is being fed to sleep. This can often lead to long-term sleeping problems for many babies.

After months of sleepless nights and exhausting days with the baby still feeding two- or three-hourly, many parents ask their GP to refer them to a baby sleep clinic. Or they purchase one or several of the many baby books on how to get your baby to sleep through the night, only to be told they got it all wrong in the first place. The real reason their baby is unable to sleep well is that he has had the wrong associations with going to sleep, i.e. feeding, rocking, patting etc.

How well your baby sleeps is very closely linked to how well he feeds, and what he associates with falling asleep. To encourage healthy sleep habits with your baby, it is important that you not only structure his feeding but you have an understanding of the sleep rhythms of young babies, so that you establish the right sleep associations from very early on.

An understanding of sleep rhythms will also help you adjust the routines to suit the individual needs of your baby, and, at times, on the occasions when it has not been possible to follow them to the letter.

## Sleep rhythms

Most of the leading experts would agree that a newborn baby will sleep approximately 16 hours a day in the first few weeks. This sleep is broken up into a series of short and longer sleeps. In the early days sleep is very much linked to the baby's need to feed little and often. It can take well up to an hour to feed, burp and change the baby, after which time he falls quickly into a deep sleep. If the baby has fed well he will often sleep through to the next feed. Over a 24-hour period, therefore, with the baby feeding 6–8 times a day and feeds lasting between 45 minutes and one hour, the baby ends up sleeping approximately 16 hours a day.

However, between the third and fourth week, the baby becomes more alert and will not fall straight into a deep sleep after feeding. This is often a time when things start to go wrong and the wrong sleep associations are developed. The anxious parents, believing that the baby should fall asleep straight after feeding, start to resort to feeding, rocking or giving the baby a dummy to induce sleep. They do not realise that it is around this age that the different stages of sleep become more apparent.

Like adults, babies drift from light sleep into a dream-like sleep known as REM sleep, then into a deep sleep. The cycle is much shorter than that of an adult, lasting approximately 45 minutes to one hour. While some babies only stir when they drift into light sleep, others will wake up fully. If the baby is due a feed, this does not create a problem. However, if it is only one hour since the baby fed, and the baby does not learn to settle himself, a real problem can develop over the months ahead if the baby is constantly assisted back to sleep by one or more of the methods I have just mentioned. Recent research has shown that all babies drift into light sleep and wake up approximately the same number of times during the night. Only the poor sleepers are unable to drift back into deep sleep, because they are used to being helped to sleep.

If you want your baby to develop good sleep habits from an early age, it is important to avoid the wrong sleep associations. My routines are structured so that your baby feeds well, never gets overtired and does not learn the wrong associations when going to sleep.

## The bedtime routine

Once your baby has regained his birth weight and is regularly putting on at least 180–240g (6–8oz) each week, you can look at establishing a regular bedtime of 6.30–7pm, and allow him to sleep past the 9pm feed, feeding him at around 10pm instead, slowly pushing forwards to 10.30pm. It is also at this stage that he should manage to go slightly longer in the night. If he feeds well at this feed, and settles at around 11–11.30pm, he will hopefully manage to sleep to between 2am and 3am. If he feeds well then and hopefully settles back within an hour, he should manage to sleep to around 6–7am, provided that he has been awake properly enough to take a full feed at the 10–10.30pm feed. During the early days, how soon they wake up after midnight is very much dependent on how awake they were at the last feed and how much they took. It is worthwhile spending some time at this feed to ensure that the baby does start to sleep a longer stretch in the night.

Establishing a good bedtime routine and getting your baby

to sleep well between 7pm and 10pm is a major factor in how quickly he will sleep through the night. A baby who feeds well at 6pm, and settles to sleep well between 7pm and 10pm, will wake up refreshed and ready to take a full feed. However, there are other factors in establishing a regular bedtime routine. The main ones are that you have structured his feeding and sleeping pattern during the day, so that he is hungry enough to take a full feed at 5–6.15pm; and that he has been awake enough during the day, so he is ready to sleep at 7pm.

I get many calls and emails from parents who are struggling to settle their babies in the evening. When a pattern of feeding on and off occurs during the evening, in most cases it has a knock-on effect of the baby not being hungry enough at the 10.30pm feed. The baby then ends up waking around 1am and usually 4–5am again, genuinely hungry.

Establishing a bedtime routine will only be possible if your baby is well fed and ready to sleep by 6.30–7pm. For example, if you allow your baby to sleep for lengthy periods in the late afternoon, he is unlikely to settle well at 7pm, even if he has fed well.

The key to encouraging your baby to sleep well at night is very dependent on what happens during the day. Once he is gaining a regular weight of at least 180–240g (6–8oz) each week, it means he is growing well. As he grows, the amount that he can take at each feed should increase, and he should gradually be able to go longer between some feeds. Ideally, this longer spell should be between 7pm and 10pm, and after the 10.30pm feed and middle-of-the-night feeds.

This will not necessarily happen automatically, which takes us back to what you may find the hardest part of the routines: waking your baby for daytime feeds at the recommended times for his age. But it is simply common sense that if your baby has fed regularly during the day, he should, as he grows, need to feed less in the night, as the amount that he takes during the day increases.

Try, whenever possible, to start the day at 7am, stick to the times I advise in the routines, and ensure that your baby takes a full feed at those times and is awake for short spells after the daytime feeds. This will help you establish a bedtime routine where your baby settles well at 7pm. Remember, if your baby feeds and settles well by 7pm and sleeps soundly until 10pm, he will be much more likely to start to sleep longer in the night after that feed. Waking him just after 10pm ensures he is wide awake and able to take a full feed at 10.30pm.

As very young babies get overtired easily, start the bedtime routine no later than 5.30pm. If your baby has not slept well at nap times you may need to start earlier. Try to keep things very calm and quiet throughout the bath, and after the bath avoid lots of eye contact and talking, so that he does not become overstimulated. Try always to do the last part of the feed in the nursery, keeping it dimly lit, so that you can quickly settle your baby in the cot before he falls into a deep sleep.

It will be difficult, but all the parents I have spoken to say that it was worth putting in the hard work in those early days, as their babies started to sleep longer and longer in the night, until they eventually make it through to that magical time of 7am.

## Early-morning waking

I have always believed that whether a child becomes an early-morning waker is very much determined by what happens during the first year. In order to avoid this problem it is crucial that the baby sleeps in a very dark room and that the mother treats any feeds before 7am as night-time feeds. They should be done with the minimum of fuss, with no talking or eye contact, and the baby should be settled back to sleep until 7am. If your baby has woken between 6am and 6.30am then leave him until 7.30am.

This approach has worked for the hundreds of babies I have helped care for, none of whom ever got up before 7am, once they were sleeping through the night. Certainly some of these babies would waken around 5–6am, and perhaps chatter or sing for a short spell, before returning to sleep.

Since the publication of the first edition of this book and my second book I have spoken to thousands of parents who have experienced problems with early-morning waking, and a further reason has become very apparent. One thing that nearly all these parents had in common is that they did not follow my advice of allowing their babies to wake up naturally. Most admitted to picking their babies up the minute they started to wake from daytime naps. Over a period of time it is not surprising that these babies came to expect the same thing to happen when they woke early in the morning.

Somewhere between eight and 12 weeks, the majority of babies do not wake up from naps immediately looking for food. This is a good time to encourage them to lie in their cot for a short time after waking. I am convinced that by doing this, along with the guidelines listed below, there will be less chance of your baby becoming an early-morning waker:

- Research shows that the chemicals in the brain work differently in the dark, preparing it for sleep. Get your baby used to sleeping in a very dark room for most of his sleep times from day one, with the door shut. Check that there are no chinks of light at the top or sides of the curtains. Even the smallest amount of light can be enough to waken the baby fully when he comes into a light sleep.
- Until they reach six months the 'Moro reflex' can be quite strong with some babies and is very obvious in the early days. The baby flings his arms and legs back in jerky movements, usually if he gets shocked, is startled by a sudden loud noise or is put down too roughly or too quickly. Hence the reason that it is often referred to as the 'startle reflex'.

  As the weeks go by and the baby becomes more relaxed, the Moro reflex is less frequent. But it can take up to seven or eight months before it disappears altogether. I have observed many babies coming into their light sleep in the middle of the night and thrashing their legs up and down hysterically because they have kicked off their covers.

For this reason I believe it is very important that a baby is tucked in very securely by his bed covers, until the Moro reflex has totally disappeared. The sheet and blankets should be placed lengthways across the width of the cot and then two rolled hand towels pushed down between the spars and the mattress. For babies who still manage to work their way up the cot, a very lightweight sleeping bag of no more than 0.5 tog can be used, along with being tucked in with a cotton sheet.

- Do not try to push your baby through the night by cutting down on his middle-of-the-night feed. Continue to give him as much as he wants in the middle of the night to ensure that he sleeps soundly to 7am. It is only when he has been sleeping through regularly to 7am for a period of time, and wakes up refusing to feed well at 7am, that you should consider cutting down the amount he is taking in the middle of the night.
- If your baby is feeding at 5–6am, treat it as a night feed. It should be done as quickly as possible in a dimly lit room without any eye contact or talking. Only change his nappy if really necessary.
- Do not drop the 10.30pm feed until your baby is established on solid food. If he goes through a growth spurt before he starts his solids, he can be offered extra milk at this feed. This reduces the chances of him waking early due to hunger.

## Your questions answered

**Q How many hours' sleep a day does my newborn baby need?**

A
- Depending on weight and whether the baby was premature, most babies need approximately 16 hours a day, broken up into a series of short and long sleeps.
- Smaller babies and premature babies tend to need more sleep, and will be more likely to doze on and off between feeds.
- Larger babies are capable of staying awake for an hour or

so and sleeping for at least one longer spell of 4–5 hours during a 24-hour period.

- By the age of one month, most babies who are feeding well and gaining weight (180–240g (6–8oz) a week) are capable of sleeping for one longer stretch of 5–6 hours between feeds.

**Q How do I make sure that the longer stretch of sleeping is always in the night and not during the day?**

A
- Follow my routines and always start your day no later than 7am, so that you have enough time to fit in all the feeds before 11pm.
- Try to keep your baby awake for at least 6–8 hours between 7am and 7pm.
- Ensure that your baby stays awake for as much of the two-hour social period as possible. Once he is awake for a total of eight hours between 7am and 7pm, he will be more likely to sleep longer in the night.
- Always distinguish between sleep and awake time. During the first few weeks, put the baby in a dark room for all sleeps.
- Do not talk to your baby or overstimulate him during the feeds between 7pm and 7am.

**Q I am trying to stick to your routines, but my four-week-old baby can only stay awake for an hour at the most after feeds. Should I be trying to make him stay awake longer?**

A
- If your baby is feeding well and gaining between 180–240g (6–8oz) per week, is sleeping well between feeds in the night and is alert for some of his awake periods during the day, he is just one of those babies who needs more sleep.
- If he is waking up more than twice in the night or staying awake for over an hour in the night despite feeding well at 11pm, try stimulating him a bit more during the day.
- While the 10.30pm feed should always be a quiet feed, a baby under three months needs to be awake for 45 minutes. A sleepy feed at this time will most certainly result in a baby being more awake around 2–3am.

- If you structure your baby's feeds and sleep times between 7am and 11pm by my routines, when your baby does cut back his sleep, it will be at the right time.

**Q The routine seems very restricting. If I go out with my four-week-old during waking time he goes straight to sleep in the buggy, which means he has slept too much.**

A
- Whether your baby is in my routine or not, during the first couple of months life is restrictive due to the amount of time spent feeding.
- By two months most babies are capable of going longer between feeds and are quicker at feeding. This makes outings easier.
- For the first two months if you plan your outings to fit around his sleep time, by eight weeks he will be able to stay awake longer when you take him out in the car or buggy.

**Q My four-week-old baby has suddenly started to wake up at nine in the evening. If I feed him then he wakes up twice in the night at 1am and 5am. I have tried encouraging him to hold out until 10.30pm, but then he is so tired he doesn't feed properly, which means he still wakes up earlier.**

A
- Around one month, the light and deep sleep becomes much more defined. I find that a lot of babies come into a very light sleep around 9pm, so ensure that the area around the nursery is not subject to loud, sudden noises and that the baby cannot hear your voice at this time.
- Breast-fed babies may need a top-up of expressed milk after the 6pm feed.
- If you have to feed him at 9pm, try to settle him with one breast or a couple of ounces, and then push the 10.30pm feed to 11.30pm. Hopefully, he will then take a full feed, which would get him through to 3.30am.

**Q I always have to wake my baby of 10 weeks for his 10.30pm feed, then he only takes 90–120ml (3–4oz) and wakes again**

**at 4am. Could I just drop the last feed and see if he goes through until 4am without that feed?**

A
- I would not advise getting rid of the feed yet, as he could wake up at 1am and then 5am, which, in effect, would be two night wakings. I have always found it best to get the baby sleeping through to 7am, and taking solids, before dropping the 10.30pm feed. This usually happens at about six months.
- Make sure he is tucked in properly; often a baby getting out of his blankets and thrashing around in his light sleep is enough to arouse him to a fully awake state. If he is not getting out of his covers, I would wait 5–10 minutes before going to him, and then I would try settling him with some water. If he settles with the water he will make up for the lost feed during the day and at his age the increased daily milk intake usually has the knock-on effect of him not needing to feed in the night. If he does not settle with the water, I would try to settle him with a small feed and try again in a couple of weeks.

# 5 Establishing the Contented Little Baby routines

The times for feeding and sleeping change 10 times during the first year of the CLB routines to ensure that the individual needs of every baby can be properly met. It is very important that you read carefully the advice and information in the feeding and sleeping chapters before you even attempt to start the routines. They will help you understand how best to use the routines so that your baby is happy, content and feeds and sleeps well.

After the birth follow the advice given in the routine for a newborn, until he has regained his birth weight and shows signs of being able to go longer between feeds. Then you can move on to the first routine for a two- to four-week baby. Gradually, when your baby shows signs of going longer between feeds and staying awake longer, you can move on to the next routine. Do not worry if your baby is not managing the routine for his age, just stick to the routine that he is happy in and continue to watch for the signs that he is content and able to go longer between feeds and stay awake longer, before moving on to the next routine.

If you are starting the routines with an older baby who has established a pattern of demand-feeding and sleeping, look through the routines and find the one nearest to the pattern he is already in. Follow that routine for a short period and then, once he is eating and feeding happily at the times in that routine, you can move on to the next routine, gradually working your way through the different routines until he eventually reaches the one suitable for his age.

## Feeding

Small babies spend a great deal of their waking time feeding. To avoid excessive night feeding, it is important to structure and establish a good daytime feeding pattern. As I have explained, in order to establish a good milk supply I believe that your baby needs to be fed little and often after the birth. The success of the CLB routines depends on the baby being woken for feeds and not being left for long spells between feeds. I recommend that in the very early days a three-hourly feeding routine be established. This time is calculated from the beginning of one feed to the beginning of the next feed. Of course, if a baby is demanding food before the recommended time I have always advised that he should be fed. But if this continues long after the milk has come in then it is important to look for reasons why your baby is not lasting longer between feeds.

Only once a baby has regained his birth weight, and continues to gain approximately 30g (1oz) a day, do I recommend that the times between feeds are extended, and only if the baby shows signs of happily going longer between feeds. By structuring your baby's feeds from early on, things should never get to a stage where he is having to cry to let you know he is hungry, as you will already be pre-empting his feeding needs.

From the very beginning it is important to differentiate between feeding, sleeping and social time. If you talk too much or overstimulate him while feeding, he could lose interest after a couple of ounces, and then may not settle well to sleep, which could result in you feeding him to sleep, which, in the long term, can create sleep problems. Also try to avoid talking on the telephone for long periods while feeding.

It is important, during the very early days, that you concentrate on the positioning of your baby on the breast to ensure that he feeds well. Do seek help from an experienced breast-feeding counsellor to make sure that you are getting the feeding position right. If you feed him in a rocking chair, do not be tempted to rock him while feeding, as he will think it is sleep time, and if he is sleepy while feeding, he will not feed so well and will need to feed again sooner. Sleepy babies are also often more prone to possetting back some of their feed.

The aim of the CLB feeding routines is to ensure that when your baby is ready to increase milk feeds, you structure his daytime feeds along with his daytime sleep. This will mean that, as soon as your baby is physically and mentally capable, he will sleep his longest spell in the night and not during the day.

## Sleep

It is essential for your baby's mental and physical development that he gets enough sleep; without the right amount he will become irritable, fretful and inconsolable. A baby who is constantly tired will not feed effectively, and therefore not sleep properly. As I have already mentioned, one of the most important things that you should try to remember in the early days is that very young babies can only stay awake for up to two hours before becoming tired. If your baby stays awake for longer than two hours he could become so exhausted that he will need a much longer sleep at his next nap time. This will have a knock-on effect, altering the rest of his routine, resulting in poor evening and night-time sleep. Therefore, it is essential that you structure the two-hourly awake period properly, so that the feeding and sleeping plan works well. In the early days some babies can only stay awake for an hour after a feed; this is fairly normal for babies who need more sleep.

To determine whether your baby is a sleepy baby or not, look at his night-time sleep. If he can only stay awake for an hour at a time during the day, but settles well in the evening, and feeds and settles quickly during the night, he is a baby who needs more sleep. He will eventually manage to stay awake for longer amounts of time provided you ensure that he is given the opportunity. You can do this by trying whenever possible to settle him in his nursery for naps, and, during his waking time, by having him in a bright, social and noisier environment. Create the contrast between naps and social time to help him learn when it's time to sleep and when it's time to play.

However, if he can only stay awake for an hour at a time during the day, but for several hours during the night, it is possible that he has got his day and night muddled up, and it is worthwhile encouraging him to stay awake more during the day. Babies learn by association. It is very important that from day one he learns the right associations, and to differentiate between feeding, playing, cuddling and sleeping.

You will also find that there are some times of the day when your baby will stay awake for two hours quite happily, and other times when he will be tired after an hour. This is perfectly normal in the early days, which is why I say that babies can stay awake for *up to* two hours – not that they *must* stay awake for two hours.

Along with the routines, the following guidelines will help your baby develop healthy sleeping habits:

- Try to keep him awake for a short spell after his day feeds.
- Do not let him sleep too long in the late afternoon.
- Do not feed him after 3.15pm, as it will put him off his night feed.
- Follow the same routine every evening; do not allow visitors in the nursery during wind-down time.
- Do not let him get overtired; allow at least one hour for the bath, feed and wind-down time.
- Do not overstimulate him or play with him after his bath.
- Do not rock him to sleep in your arms; try to settle him in his cot before he goes into a deep sleep.
- If you use a dummy to wind him down, remove it before you put him in his cot.
- If he falls asleep on the breast or bottle, arouse him slightly before settling him in his cot.

## Playing

All babies love to be cuddled, and talked and sung to. Research also shows that even very small babies like to look at simple books and interesting toys. For your baby to enjoy these things, it is important that you do them at the right time. The best time is usually approximately one hour after he is awake and has been fed. He should never be played with or overstimulated 20 minutes prior to his nap. Try to imagine how you would feel if you were just drifting off to sleep and someone came into the room and wanted to laugh and joke with you. I doubt you would be too happy about it, so try to respect that your baby needs the same quiet time before he goes off to sleep.

Pay particular attention to what toys you get your baby used to in his cot. I find it a great help to divide toys and books into wake-up and wind-down ones. Musical cot mobiles and colourful baby gyms, plus black and white cloth cot books are all excellent for keeping young babies interested for short spells, during social time, as are postcards and posters that show single objects or faces. Use these toys only at social times and two or three different, less stimulating toys for wind-down times.

Babies have very short concentration spans; constantly talking and handling a baby during the social time can often result in him becoming overstimulated. It's important to take the cue from your baby as to how much stimulation he can handle. Even from a very young age, babies should be encouraged to occupy themselves for short periods and have freedom to move. This is much more likely to happen if the baby is allowed to lie on his playmat or under his cot mobile, as he will be able to kick and move around more than when he is being held.

## Cuddling

Babies need lots of cuddling, but it should always be done when your baby needs it, not when you need it. A baby needs energy to grow, so it is important that you do not overhandle his small body and exhaust him. While all babies need to be nurtured, they are not toys. Differentiate the type of cuddle during his playtime from that of wind-down time. Wind-down cuddling should be about closeness of bodies. It is important that your baby is not cuddled to sleep while feeding. After one hour of being awake and fed he should be happy to spend a little time amusing himself; if you constantly cuddle him during playtime, he will be less likely to respond to the cuddles that would normally help settle him for his nap. When cuddling him during the wind-down time, do not talk and avoid eye contact, as it can overstimulate him and result in him becoming overtired and not settling. Instead, just enjoy that peaceful connection and closeness that you feel with him.

## Structuring the milk feeds during the first year

During the first few weeks, regardless of whether babies are breast- or formula-fed, very few can manage a strict four-hourly feeding pattern, and the aim of the CLB feeding routines is to ensure that the individual needs of all babies can be met. That is why I recommend that babies are fed three-hourly in the early days, and only when they have regained their birth weight and are gaining approximately 30g (1oz) a day should they be left to go longer for feeds. By two weeks, if your baby has regained his birth weight and weighs over 3.2kg (7lb), he should manage to last 3–4 hours between some feeds, provided he is getting a full feed at the times stated in the routines. By structuring feeds in the early days you can achieve several slots of three-hour feeding and some of a four-hour stretch. If you structure his feeds according to the routines, the four-hour stretch between feeds should always happen between 10am and 2pm and 7pm to 7am. This would mean that a baby who fed at 6pm should get to 10pm, then feed again around 2–3am, then get to 5/6–7am.

Remember that the three-hour stretch between feeds is timed from the beginning of one feed to the beginning of the next; a baby starting to feed at 7am would then need to start his next feed at 10am. However, if you feel your baby is genuinely hungry before his next feed is due, as I have mentioned earlier, he must be fed – but it is also advisable to get to the root of the problem as to why he is not taking a full feed at the times stated in the routines. If you are breast-feeding, it may be that he needs longer on the second breast; if you are bottle-feeding, it may be that he needs an extra ounce at some feeds.

Between the second and fourth week, most babies who are gaining 180–240g (6–8oz) each week are able to last slightly longer after one feed – usually four and a half to five hours. If you structure your baby's feeds, this will automatically be at the right time, i.e. between 11pm and 7am.

If your baby has been demand-fed and you are attempting to put him into a routine, I would advise that you look at the early routines and put him into a routine that seems nearest to his demand-fed pattern. For example, a nine-week-old baby may need to start on the two- to four-week schedule. When he is happy in that routine, you should be able to work your way through the next two sets of routines within 7–10 days. By the time he reaches 12 weeks, he should be happily feeding at the times stated in the routine for his age. However, although it may take slightly longer for him to sleep through the night, the important thing is that he is only feeding once in the night and gradually increasing the length of time he sleeps from his last feed, over a period of several weeks. Once the baby starts to sleep longer in the night, it is important to keep a close eye on how you structure feeds, as things can go wrong, particularly if you have been *too* strict. Remember the whole key to the CLB feeding routines is that they are flexible and that no baby should ever be forced to go longer before feeding than he is physically capable of.

The following extract is from the diary of a mother with a five-week-old baby going approximately four hours between feeds. It shows how quickly things can go wrong, when a strict four-hourly routine is followed.

| | | | | | | |
|---|---|---|---|---|---|---|
| **Tues** | 3am | 7am | 11am | 3pm | 7pm | 11pm |
| **Wed** | 3am | 7am | 11am | 3pm | 7pm | 11pm |
| **Thurs** | 4am | 8am | 12pm | 4pm | 8pm | 12am |
| **Fri** | 5am | 9am | 1pm | 5pm | 9pm | 11pm |
| **Sat** | 2am | 6am | 10am | 2pm | 6pm | 10pm |
| **Sun** | 2am | 6am | 10am | 2pm | 6pm | 10pm |

Aware that the feeding pattern was going haywire, the mother tried to get it back on track on the Friday night by waking the baby up at 11pm. This did not work, as the baby had taken a full feed at 9pm and was not hungry. It resulted in such a poor feed that the baby woke up at 2am needing a full feed, which meant a total backtrack on night feeding. Even if the mother had managed to settle the baby at 9pm with a smaller feed, it is unlikely the baby would have fed any better. The baby had only been asleep for one hour so it would have been very difficult to wake him up enough to feed properly.

As I mentioned earlier, the easiest way to keep your baby on track is to wake him at 7am. Once he is sleeping to 5am or 6am, he should be offered a top-up feed at 7am or 7.30am. This method will not only keep the rest of your feeds on track, but ensure that your baby's sleeping is kept on track as well and that he is ready to go to bed at 7pm.

The following advice will also ensure that your baby sleeps through the night as soon as he is physically able, and prepare him for the introduction of solids and the eventual reduction of milk feeds.

## Understanding the routines for feeding

### The 6–7am feed

- Depending on what time he fed in the night, your baby will probably wake up between 6am and 7am, but he should always be woken at 7am regardless. Remember that one of the main keys to getting your baby to sleep through the night is to ensure that once he is physically capable of bigger feeds, he takes his daily requirements between 7am and 11pm.
- Regardless of whether he is breast- or bottle-fed, the only way to keep a baby in a good routine is to begin the day at 7am. Once he is sleeping through the night, he should be at his hungriest at this feed.

- During growth spurts, breast-fed babies should be given longer on the breast to ensure that their increased needs are met. If you have been expressing you can reduce this by 30ml (1oz) to ensure that his needs are immediately met. If you have not expressed, you can still follow the feeding times from the routine for your baby's age, but you will have to top him up with a short breast-feed before his daytime naps. If you do this for a week or so, this should help increase your milk supply. A sign that this has happened is that your baby will sleep well at the naps, and not be so interested in the next feed. Once this happens you can gradually decrease the length of time that you top-up for, until you are back on your original feeding schedule. A formula-fed baby should have his feeds increased by 30ml (1oz) when he is regularly draining his bottle.

*By seven months*

- If your baby is eating a full breakfast of cereal, fruit and perhaps small pieces of toast, you should aim to cut back the amount offered to him from the breast or bottle. Try to divide the milk between a drink and with the cereal. Always try to encourage him to take at least 150–180ml (5–6 oz) before he is given his solids.
- If you are still breast-feeding, gradually reduce the time he is on the first breast, then give him his solids and, finally, a further short feed from the second breast. Keep a very close watch that you do not allow him to increase his solids so much that he cuts back too much on his breast-feed.
- Your baby still needs a minimum of 600ml (20oz) a day, inclusive of milk used in cooking or on cereal, divided between 3–4 milk feeds.

*By ten months*

- If your baby is formula-fed, try to encourage him to take all his milk from a beaker. Ensure that you still offer milk at the start of the meal. Once he has taken 150–180ml (5–6oz) of his milk, offer him some cereal. Then offer him the remainder of his milk again.

- It is important that he has at least 180–240 ml (6–8oz) of milk divided between the beaker and the breakfast cereal.
- If you are still breast-feeding, offer him first the breast then the solids, then offer him the breast again.
- Your baby needs a minimum of 540ml (18oz) a day, inclusive of milk used in cooking or on cereal, divided between two or three milk feeds.

### The 10–11am feed

- During the first few weeks, the majority of babies who have fed between 6am and 7am will wake looking for a feed around 10am. Even if your baby does not do this it is important that you wake him. Remember that the aim is to ensure that your baby feeds regularly during the day so that he only needs to wake once for a feed between 11pm and 6–7am.
- In the early days, many babies would happily sleep 4–5 hours between feeds during the day. Regardless of whether a baby is breast-fed or bottle-fed, within a very short period of time this usually leads to several night-time feeds as the baby attempts to make up for his daily nutritional needs. It also puts him at possible risk of dehydration.
- Too few feeds during the day in the early weeks also does little to help establish a good milk supply for a breast-feeding mother, and feeding several times a night soon exhausts the mother so much that her milk supply is reduced even further.
- Around six weeks, your baby may show signs of being happy to go longer from the 7am feed, and the 10am feed can gradually be pushed to 10.30am. However, a baby who is feeding at 5am or 6am and being topped up at 7.30am would probably still need to feed at 10am, as would the baby who has too small a feed at 7am.
- Once he is sleeping through the night, or taking only a small

feed in the night, he should have the biggest feed of the day at 6.45–7am. If he feeds well, he should be happy to last until 11am before needing another feed. However, if you feed him before he really needs it, he may not feed well and, as a result, may sleep poorly at the lunchtime nap. This will have a knock-on effect so that each subsequent feed and nap has to be given earlier and may result in the baby waking up at 6am or earlier the following morning.

- This feed would be the next one to be increased during growth spurts.

*By six to seven months*

- When your baby is eating breakfast, you can start to make this feed later, eventually settling somewhere between 11.30am and 12 noon. This will be the pattern for three meals a day at the end of six months, at which stage the milk feed will be replaced with a drink of well-diluted juice or water from a beaker.
- It is important that you introduce the tier system of feeding so that he gradually cuts back on the milk feed and increases his solids.
- Some babies simply refuse to cut back on this milk feed. If you find that your baby is one, please refer to page 219 for suggestions on how to deal with this.

*By seven months*

- When your baby is on a proper balanced diet of solids, which includes protein with lunch, it is important that this feed should be replaced with a drink of water or well-diluted juice. Formula milk given with a protein meal can reduce the iron absorption by up to 50 per cent.
- Give the baby most of his solids before his drink so he doesn't fill up with liquid first.

## The 2.30pm feed

- During the first few months, make this feed smaller so that your baby feeds really well at the 5–6.15pm feed, the exception being if your baby doesn't sleep well at lunchtime and needs feeding earlier with a top-up at 2.30pm. If, for some reason, the baby feeds badly at the 10am feed or was fed earlier, increase this feed accordingly so that he maintains his daily milk quota.
- If your baby is very hungry and regularly drains the bottle at this feed then you can give him the full amount, provided he does not take less at the next feed.
- For breast-fed babies, allow longer on the breast if he is not managing to get through happily to the next feed.

*By eight months*

- When your baby is having three full solid meals a day and his lunchtime milk feed has been replaced with water or well-diluted juice, you will probably need to increase this feed so that he is getting his daily milk quota in three milk feeds.
- However, if he cuts back on the last milk feed of the day, it would be advisable to keep this milk feed smaller and make up the daily quota by using milk in cereals and cooking.
- Your baby still needs a minimum of 600ml (20oz) a day, inclusive of milk used on breakfast cereal and in cooking.

*By nine to twelve months*

- Bottle-fed babies should be given their milk from a beaker at this stage, which should automatically result in a decrease in the amount they drink.
- If this is not the case and your baby starts to lose interest in his morning or evening feed, you could cut right back on this feed. If he is getting 540ml (18oz) of milk a day (inclusive of milk used in cooking and on cereal), plus a full balanced diet of solids, you could cut this feed altogether.

- By one year of age your baby needs a minimum of 350ml (12oz) a day, inclusive of milk used in cooking and on cereal.

**The 6 –7pm feed**

- It is important that your baby always has a good feed at this time if you want him to settle well between 7pm and 10pm.
- He should not be fed milk after 3.15pm, as it could put him off taking a really good feed at this time.
- In the first few weeks, this feed is split between 5pm and 6.15pm so that the baby does not get too frantic during his bath. Once your baby has slept through the night for two weeks, the 5pm feed can be dropped. I would not recommend dropping the split feed until this happens, as a larger feed at 6.15pm could result in your baby taking even less at the last feed, resulting in an earlier waking time. With many of the babies that I cared for, I kept giving them a split feed until solids were introduced to ensure that they were getting enough milk during the day. Once you eliminate the 5pm feed and your baby is taking a full feed after the bath, he could cut down dramatically on his last feed of the day, which could result in an early waking.
- Breast-fed babies not settling at 7pm should be offered a top-up of expressed milk. Your milk supply may well be low at this time of the day.

*By four to five months*

- If your baby has started solids early, he should be given most of his milk before his solids, as milk is still the most important form of nutrition at this age.
- Most babies would be taking a full breast- or formula-feed at this age.
- If he is weaned and very tired at this feed and you are struggling to get him to take all of his milk feed plus any solids you have been advised to introduce, adjust the feeding times. Try giving two-thirds of each milk feed at around 5.30pm followed by his solids, then delay his bath to around

6.25pm. After the bath he can then be offered the remainder of his milk feed. If formula feeding, it is advisable to make up two separate bottles to ensure that the milk is fresh.
- A breast-fed baby who has reached five months, is weaned and is now starting to wake up before 10.30pm may not be getting enough at this time. Try giving a full breast-feed at 5.30pm followed by the solids, with a bath at 6.15pm, followed by a top-up of expressed milk or formula after the bath. A baby who is not weaned would more than likely need to continue to have a split milk feed at 5–6.15pm until solids are introduced.

*By six to seven months*

- Most babies will now be having tea at 5pm followed by a full breast-feed or a full formula-feed. Once solids are established and the 10.30pm feed is dropped, you may find that if you are breast-feeding, your baby starts to wake earlier. I would suggest that if this happens you should offer a top-up of expressed milk to ensure that he settles well at 7pm and sleeps through until the morning.

*By ten to twelve months*

- Bottle-fed babies should be taking all of their milk from a beaker at one year. Babies who continue to feed from a bottle after this age are more prone to feeding problems, as they continue to take large amounts, which takes the edge off their appetite for solids.
- Start encouraging your baby to take some of his milk from a beaker at 10 months, so that by one year he is happy to take all of his last feed from a beaker.

## The 10–11pm feed

- I strongly advise that parents of breast-fed babies should introduce bottles of either expressed milk or formula at this feed, no later than the second week. This will help you share the feeding responsibilities with a partner or other carer.

- This also helps to avoid the common problem of a baby refusing to take a bottle at a later stage.
- A totally breast-fed baby under three months who continues to wake up between 2am and 3am and shows no sign of going a longer spell in the night, may not be getting enough to eat at this time, as the breast milk supply is often at its lowest at this time of day.
- If you choose to top up with expressed milk or formula rather than completely replacing the feed with a full bottle-feed, it is essential that you ensure that your baby has completely emptied the breast before he is offered the top-up feed.
- It is easier to tell whether formula-fed babies are getting enough to eat at this feed. If you always increase the day feeds during your baby's growth spurts, he will probably never require more than 180ml (6oz) at this feed. However, some babies who weighed more than 4.5kg (10lb) at birth may reach a stage where they need more than this, until they are well established on solids.
- Refer to page 62 for guidelines on how much formula your baby needs to drink every day.

*By three to four months*

- If your baby has slept through the night until 7am for at least two weeks, then you can bring this feed forward by 10 minutes every three nights, until your baby is sleeping from 10pm to 6.45–7am.
- If your baby is totally breast-fed and is still waking up early in the night, despite being topped up with expressed milk at the late feed, it may be worthwhile talking to your health visitor about replacing the late breast-feeds with formula-feeds. Most formula-fed babies will be taking 210–240ml (7–8oz) a feed 4–5 times a day.
- If a formula-fed baby is not sleeping through the night at this age, it may be because he needs a little extra at this feed, and

even if it means he cuts back on his morning feed, it may be worthwhile offering him an extra ounce or two.

- Some babies simply refuse this feed at 3–4 months. If your baby is feeding well from the breast four times a day and your health visitor is happy with his weight gain, you can just drop this feed. However, if you find that he starts to wake earlier again and will not settle back to sleep within 10 minutes or so, you would have to assume that it could be hunger and feed him. You may then have to consider re-introducing the 10.30pm feed until he is weaned and established on solids.
- If your baby is waking twice in the night (i.e. 2am and 5am) or is not sleeping past 5am, you can try waking the baby at 9.45pm for this feed. Ensure he is wide awake either by changing his nappy, or by letting him have a kick around on his mat. Turn all the lights on. He should be feeding by 10pm. Try then to keep him up until 11pm by changing him or playing (whichever you didn't do at 9.45pm). Top him up just before he goes down at 11pm. By ensuring he is awake for longer at this feed and splitting it, he should only wake once in the night. Once this is established and he is going for a longer spell at night, you can slowly move the beginning of this feed back to 10/10.15pm.

*By four to seven months*

- The majority of babies should be capable of sleeping through the night from their last feed at this age, provided they are having their daily intake of milk between 7am and 11pm.
- A baby who is being exclusively breast-fed may only manage to get through to around 5am until he is weaned.
- Once your baby has been weaned and is established on three solid meals a day, this last feed should gradually reduce automatically. This will depend on how much solid food your baby is taking once he is aged between six and seven

months. If you have been advised to wean your baby earlier than six months, you should find that you could drop this feed fairly quickly once he reaches this age. A baby who did not start solids until the recommended age of six months may still need this feed until he reaches seven months. By this time, provided the baby is taking enough milk and solids during the day, you should be able to gradually reduce the amount he takes and then eliminate it altogether.

### The 2–3am feed

- Newborn babies need to feed little and often during the first week so when they wake it is best to assume that they are hungry and feed them.
- A newborn baby should never be allowed to go longer then three hours between feeds during the day and four hours between feeds in the night. **This time is three hours from the beginning of one feed to the beginning of the next**.
- Once your baby has regained his birth weight, he should start to settle into the two- to four-week routine. Provided he feeds well between 10pm and 11pm, he should manage to sleep to nearer 2am.

*By four to six weeks*

- Most babies weighing over 3.2kg (7lb) at birth and gaining a regular 180–240kg (6–8oz) each week are capable of lasting a longer stretch between feeds during the night, as long as:
  (a) The baby is definitely over 4kg (9lb) in weight and taking his daily allowance of milk in the five feeds between 7am and 11pm.
  (b) The baby is not sleeping more than four and a half hours between 7am and 7pm.

*By six to eight weeks*

- If your baby is over 4kg (9lb) in weight and gaining 180–240g (6–8oz) each week but is still waking between 2am and 3am, despite taking a good feed at 10.30pm, try to settle him with some cool, boiled water. If he refuses to settle then you will have to feed him, but it would be advisable to refer to Chapter 8 to check for possible reasons why he is not going longer in the night.

- If the baby does settle, he will probably wake up again around 5am, at which time you can give him a full feed, followed by a top-up at 7–7.30am. This will help keep him on track with his feeding and sleeping pattern for the rest of the day.
- Within a week, babies usually sleep until nearer 5am, gradually increasing their sleep time until 7am. During this stage, when your baby is taking a top-up at 7–7.30am instead of a full feed, he may not manage to get through to 10.45–11am for his next feed. You may need to give him half his feed at 10am followed by the remainder at 10.45–11am, followed by a top-up just before he goes down for his lunchtime nap, to ensure that he does not wake up early from the nap.

*By three to four months*

- Both breast-fed and bottle-fed babies should be able to go for one long spell during the night by this age, provided they are getting their daily intake of milk between 6–7am and 10–11pm.
- Your baby should be sleeping no more than three hours between 7am and 7pm.
- If your baby insists on waking before 4/5am in the night, refuses cool boiled water and will not settle without feeding, keep a very detailed diary listing exact times and amounts of feeding and times of daytime naps. A baby who cuts right back on his 7am feed could be waking out of habit rather than hunger.
- Some breast-fed babies may still genuinely need to feed in the night if they are not getting enough at their last feed. If you are not already doing so, it is worth considering a top-up feed of expressed milk or formula, or a replacement formula feed at the 10.30pm feed.

- Whether you are breast-feeding or bottle-feeding, if your baby's weight gain is good, you are convinced he is waking up from habit and he refuses cool boiled water, try leaving it for 15–20 minutes before going to him. Some babies will grumble on and off then settle themselves back to sleep.
- A baby of this age may still be waking up in the night because he is getting out of his covers. Tuck him in using two rolled-up towels wedged between the mattress and the spars of the cot to keep the sheet firm.

*By four to five months*

If your baby reaches five months and is still waking in the night, you probably need to persevere with his routine, paying increased attention to the timings of the feeds and the amount of daytime sleep he is getting. If you feel that he is showing signs that he is ready to be weaned, consult your health visitor or GP for advice as to whether he should begin earlier than the recommended six months (see Chapter 7 for more details).

*Milk feeding chart for the first year*

| Age | Times |
|---|---|
| **2-4 weeks** | 2-3am 6-7am 10-10.30am 2-2.30am 5pm 6-6.30pm 10-11pm |
| **4-6 weeks** | 3-4am 6-7am 10.30-11am 2-2.30pm 5pm 6-6.30pm 10-11pm |
| **6-8 weeks** | 4-5am 7.30am 10.45-11am 2-2.30pm 6-6.30pm 10-11pm |
| **8-10 weeks** | 5-6am 7.30am 11am 2-2.30pm 6-6.30pm 10-11pm |
| **10-12 weeks** | 7am 11am 2-2.30pm 6-6.30pm 10-11pm |
| **3-4 months** | 7am 11am 2-2.30pm 6-6.30pm 10-10.30pm |
| **4-5 months** | 7am 11am 2-2.30pm 6-6.30pm 10pm |
| **5-6 months** | 7am 11.30am 2-2.30pm 6-6.30pm |
| **6-7 months** | 7am 2-2.30pm 6-6.30pm |
| **7-8 months** | 7am 2-2.30pm 6-6.30pm |
| **8-9 months** | 7am 2-2.30pm 6-6.30pm |
| **9-10 months** | 7am 5pm 6.30-7pm |
| **10-12 months** | 7am 5pm 6.30-7pm |

# Structuring daytime sleep during the first year

The whole aim of the CLB routines is to ensure that the timings of feeds fit in with your baby's daily sleep requirements. A baby who does not feed well during the day, will not sleep well during the day; and to ensure good night-time sleep for your baby it is essential that you structure his daytime sleep. Too much can result in night-time wakings. Too little can result in an overtired, irritable baby who has difficulty settling himself to sleep, and who falls asleep only when he is totally exhausted.

When following the routines it is important to remember that they are guidelines to help you decide just how long your baby can stay awake, before he needs to nap. In the routines I stress that most babies in the early days can stay awake happily for **up to two hours** before needing a nap. I do not say that they *must* stay awake for the full two hours, only that it is important that they do not stay awake longer than two hours, if overtiredness is to be avoided. So if, during the early days, you find that your baby is only staying awake for an hour or an hour and a half at a time, you do not need to worry as he is obviously a baby that needs more sleep, and as he grows he will start to stay awake longer.

Of course, if you have a baby who is only staying awake an hour at a time during the day, and partying for several hours in the night, this is a different matter, and you may have to try harder to encourage him to stay awake longer during the day if excessive night-time waking is to be avoided. Please refer to page 85 for details on how to deal with this problem.

### The importance of nap times

Infant sleep expert Marc Weissbluth (see page 197) has carried out extensive research into the nap patterns of more than 200 children. He says that napping is one of the healthy habits that sets the stage for good overall sleep and explains that a nap offers the baby a break from stimuli and allows him to recharge for further activity. Charles Schaefer PhD, Professor of Psychology at Fairleigh Dickinson University in Teaneck, New Jersey, supports this and says: 'Naps structure the day, shape both the baby's and the mother's moods, and offer the only opportunity for Mom to relax or accomplish a few tasks.'

Several leading experts on child care are in agreement that naps are essential to a baby's brain development. John Herman PhD, infant sleep expert and Associate Professor of Psychology and Psychiatry at the University of Texas, says: 'If activities are being scheduled to the detriment of sleep, it's a mistake. Parents should come after sleeping and eating.' I couldn't agree more.

By 3–4 months, most babies are capable of sleeping 12 hours at night (with a sleepy feed at 10pm), provided their daytime sleep is no more than three to three and a half hours, divided between two or three naps a day. If you want your baby to sleep from 7–7.30pm to 7–7.30am, it is very important you structure these naps so that he has his longest nap at midday, with two shorter ones in the morning and late afternoon. While it may be more convenient to let your baby have a longer nap in the morning followed by a shorter nap in the afternoon, this can lead to problems as he gets older.

Once he reduces his daytime sleep naturally, he is most likely to cut back on his late-afternoon nap. His longest nap of the day would then be in the morning. By late afternoon he will be exhausted and need to go to bed by 6.30pm. This could result in him waking up at 6am. If you manage to get him to have a nap in the late afternoon, you could then be faced with the problem of him not settling well at 7–7.30pm.

## Understanding the sleeping routine

### Morning nap

Most babies are ready for a nap approximately two hours from the time they wake up in the morning. This should always be a short nap, around 45 minutes to one hour. Between 12 and 18 months, they may reduce the time of the nap or cut it out altogether. You will know your baby is ready to drop this nap when he starts taking a long time to settle, and ends up only sleeping 10–15 minutes of his 45-minute nap. If this continues for a couple of weeks and he manages to get through to his lunchtime nap happily, cut out the morning nap altogether. It is very important that you always start to wake him up after the 45-minute period, even if he has only slept for 10 minutes. If you allow him to sleep past this time, you will not know whether he is ready to drop the nap. It could also cause him to sleep too little at his lunchtime nap, which could result in the problems that I discussed earlier.

*Six weeks onwards*

Until a proper sleep pattern has been established, try to ensure that this nap takes place in his nursery, in the dark, with the door shut. Once a proper daytime routine has been established, this nap could at times be taken in the buggy or car seat if you have to go out, but do remember to wake him after the 45 minutes.

If he is awake at 7am, he may still need a short nap of 30 minutes at 9.30am. If you find that he is only sleeping 10–15 minutes and is getting through happily to his lunchtime nap, you could cut this nap out altogether. If he sleeps to 8am, he should be able to get through to his lunchtime nap without the morning nap.

### Lunchtime nap

This should always be the longest sleep of the day. By establishing a good lunchtime nap, you will ensure that your baby is not too tired to enjoy afternoon activities, and that bedtime is relaxed and happy. Recent research shows that a nap between noon and 2pm is deeper and more refreshing than a later nap because it coincides with the baby's natural dip in alertness. As I explained earlier, allowing a longer nap in the morning, followed by a shorter one at this time, will, in turn, affect the rest of his sleep, which can result in an early-morning awakening.

Most babies will need a sleep of two to two and a half hours until they are 18 months to two years of age, when it will gradually reduce to one to one and half hours. By three years of age, they may not need a sleep after lunch, but they should always be encouraged to have some quiet time in their room. Otherwise, they are likely to get very hyperactive by late afternoon, which can affect the night sleep.

*Six weeks onwards*

If your baby is sleeping the full 45 minutes in the morning, he should be woken after two hours. If, for some reason, his morning nap was much shorter, then you could allow him two and a half hours. If your baby develops a problem with his night-time sleep, do not make the mistake of letting him sleep longer during the day.

In the early days, a lunchtime nap may sometimes go wrong and your baby will refuse to go back to sleep. Obviously, he cannot make it through from 1pm to 4pm happily. I find the best way to deal with this is to allow 30 minutes after the 2.30pm feed, then a further 30 minutes at 4.30pm. This should stop him becoming overtired and irritable, and get things back on track so that he goes to sleep well at 7pm. See page 226 for more in-depth problem-solving.

*Six months onwards*

If your baby is on three meals a day, you should be aiming to move the morning nap from 9am to 9.30am and you will most likely need to adjust the lunchtime nap to 12.30pm-2.30pm. If he is sleeping less than two hours at lunchtime, check that his morning nap between 7am and 12 noon is no more than 30 minutes.

*Twelve months onwards*

If your baby has difficulty in settling for the nap, or is waking up after one to one and a half hours, you might have to cut the morning nap right back or get rid of it altogether. Do not let him sleep after 2.30pm if you want him to go to sleep at 7pm.

### Late-afternoon nap

This is the shortest nap of the three, and the one the baby should drop first. It is essential that your baby learn to sleep in places other than his cot so it is a good idea occasionally to let him catnap in his buggy or chair at this time. This also allows you the freedom to get out and about.

*Three months onwards*

If you want your baby to go to sleep at 7pm, he should never sleep more than 45 minutes at this nap, and he should always be awake by 5pm, regardless of how long or short his sleep was. Most babies who are sleeping well at the other two naps will gradually cut back on this sleep until they cut it out altogether. If, for some reason his lunchtime nap was cut short, you would need to allow him a short sleep now, but ensure that his daily total does not exceed the amount needed for his age.

## Adjusting the routines

### Birth to six months

I have tried many different routines over the years and, without exception, I have found the 7am to 7pm routine to be the one in which tiny babies and young infants are happiest. It fits in with their natural sleep rhythms and their need to feed little and often. I urge parents to try and stick to the original routine whenever possible. Once your baby reaches the age of six months, is on four or five feeds a day and needs less sleep, it is possible to change the routine without affecting your baby's natural needs for the right amount of sleep and number of feeds.

Up to the age of six months, the following points should be noted when planning a routine:

- In the very early weeks, to avoid more than one waking in the night, you must fit in at least five feeds before midnight. This can only be done if your baby starts his day at 6am or 7am.
- An 8am to 8pm routine in the first few weeks would mean your baby would end up feeding twice between midnight and 7am.

### Six months onwards

From six months, when your baby has started solids and you have dropped the 10.30pm feed, it is easier to adjust the routine. If your baby has been sleeping regularly to 7am, it could be possible to change to a 7.30am or 8am start, and push the rest of the routine forward. Your baby would obviously need to go to sleep later in the evenings. If you want your baby to sleep later but still go to bed at 7pm, try the following:

- Cut right back on the morning nap, so that your baby is ready to go to bed at 12–12.30pm.
- Allow a nap of no longer than two hours at lunchtime and no late afternoon nap.

### Out and about

In the first few weeks, most young babies will go to sleep the minute they are in the car or the buggy. If possible, try to organise shopping trips during the sleep times so that the routine is not too disrupted. Once the routine is established and your baby is nearer eight weeks, you will find that you are able to go out more without him falling asleep the whole time.

If you are planning a day visit to friends, depending on the length of the visit, you can usually work it into the routine by travelling between 9am and 10am, or 1pm and 2pm. By the time you arrive at the destination, the baby will be due for a feed and can be kept awake. Likewise, by making the return journey between 4pm and 5pm or after 7pm, you should manage to keep things on track.

Guide to sleep required during the first year

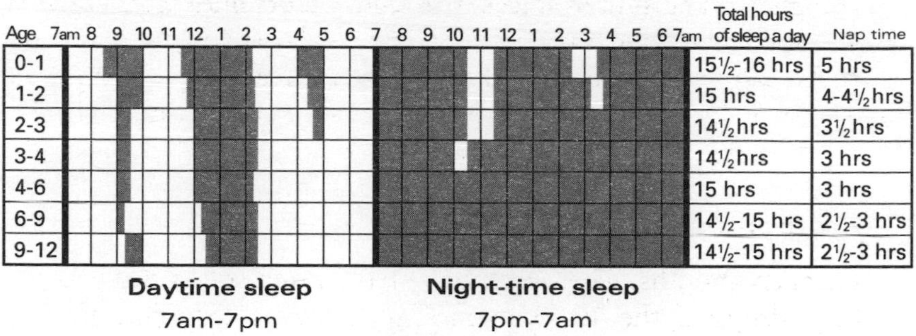

# The CLB routines for the first year 6

Please note that if you are a parent of twins, I have adapted all of the CLB routines for twins and they are collected together in *A Contented House with Twins*. This book covers many aspects of life in the first year which are unique to twins and was written in response to many requests from the mothers and fathers of twin babies.

## Routine for a breast-feeding baby at one week

| **Feed Times** | **Nap times between 7am and 7pm** |
|---|---|
| 7am | 8.30am–10am |
| 10am–11.15am | 11.30am–2pm |
| 2pm | 3.30pm–5pm |
| 5pm | |
| 6.15pm | |
| 10pm–11.15pm | **Maximum daily sleep:** 5½ hours |
| Expressing times: 6.45am, 10.45am | |

**7am**

- Baby should be awake, nappy changed and feeding no later than 7am.
- He needs 25–35 minutes on the full breast, then offer 10–15 minutes on the second breast after you have expressed 60–90ml (2–3oz).

- If he fed at 5am or 6am, offer 20–25 minutes from the second breast after expressing approximately 90ml (3oz).
- **Do not feed after 8am, as it will put baby off his next feed.** He can stay awake for up to one and a half hours.

**8am**
- Make sure you get some breakfast yourself – aim for some cereal, toast and a drink no later than 8am.

**8.15am**
- Baby should start to get a bit sleepy by this time. **Even if he does not show signs, he will be getting tired, so take him to his room now.** Check his nappy and draw sheet and close the curtains.

**8.30am**
- **Before he is asleep or before he goes into a deep sleep, settle baby in his cot, fully swaddled (see page 22) in the dark with the door shut, no later than 9am.** He needs a sleep of no longer than one and a half hours.
- This is a good time to wash and sterilise any bottles and expressing equipment.

**9.45am**
- Open the curtains and unswaddle the baby so that he can wake up naturally.
- Prepare things for top-and-tailing and dressing.

**10am**
- **Baby must be fully awake now regardless of how long he slept.**
- He should be given 25–35 minutes from the breast he last fed on while you drink a large glass of water.
- Lay him in his Moses basket or cot so he can have a good kick and doesn't become too sleepy, while you prepare equipment for expressing.

**10.45am**

- Express 60ml (2oz) from the second breast.
- Wash and dress baby, remembering to cream all his creases.

**11am**

- He should then be offered 15–20 minutes from the breast you have just expressed from.

**11.20am**

- Baby should start to get a bit sleepy by this time. **Even if he does not show the signs, he will be getting tired, so take him to his room now.**
- Check the draw sheet and change his nappy.
- Close the curtains and settle baby once he is drowsy, fully swaddled and in the dark with the door shut, no later than 11.30am.
- If he doesn't settle within 10 minutes, offer him 10 minutes from the fullest breast. Do this in the dark with no talking or eye contact.

**11.30am–2pm**

- Baby needs a nap of no longer than two and a half hours from the time he went down.
- **If he wakes up after 45 minutes, check the swaddle, but do not talk to him or turn the lights on.**
- **Allow 10 minutes for him to resettle himself;** if he's still unsettled offer him half his 2pm feed and try to settle him back to sleep until 2pm.

**12 noon**

- Wash and sterilise expressing equipment, then you should have lunch and rest before the next feed.

**2pm**

- **Baby must be awake and feeding no later than 2pm, regardless of how long he has slept.**
- Open the curtains, unswaddle him and allow him to wake naturally. Change his nappy.

- Give him 25–35 minutes from the breast he last fed on. If he is still hungry offer 10–15 minutes from the other breast while you drink a large glass of water.
- **Do not feed him after 3.15pm, as it will put him off his next feed.**
- **It is very important that he is fully awake now until 3.30pm, so he goes down well at 7pm;** if he was very alert in the morning, he may be more sleepy now. Do not put too many clothes on him, as extra warmth might make him drowsy.

**3.30pm**
- Change baby's nappy. This is a good time to take him for a walk to ensure that he sleeps well, and is refreshed for his bath and next feed.
- **Baby should not sleep after 5pm if you want him to go down well at 7pm.**

**5pm**
- **Baby must be fully awake and feeding no later than 5pm.**
- Give him a good 25–30 minutes on the breast he last fed on.
- **It is very important that he is not dozy while feeding and that he waits for the other breast until after his bath.**

**5.45pm**
- **If baby has been very wakeful during the day or didn't nap well between 3.30pm and 5pm, he may need to start his bath early.**
- Allow him a good kick without his nappy while preparing things needed for his bath and bedtime.

**6pm**
- Baby must start his bath no later than 6pm, and be massaged and dressed by 6.15pm.

**6.15pm**
- **Baby must be feeding no later than 6.15pm;** this should be done in the nursery with dim lights and no talking or eye contact.

- If he did not empty the first breast at 5pm, give him 5–10 minutes on it before putting him on the full breast. Allow a good 20–25 minutes on the full breast.
- **It is very important that baby is in bed two hours from when he last awoke.**

**7pm**

- **When he becomes drowsy, settle him fully swaddled and in the dark, with the door shut, no later than 7pm.**
- If he doesn't settle within 10–15 minutes, offer him 10 minutes from the fullest breast. Do this in the dark with no talking or eye contact.

**8pm**

- **It is very important that you have a really good meal and a rest before the next feed or expressing.**

**9.45pm**

- Turn the lights on fully and unswaddle baby so that he can wake up naturally. Allow at least 10 minutes before feeding to ensure that he is fully awake, so that he can feed well.
- Lay out things for the nappy change, plus a spare draw sheet, muslin and swaddle blanket in case they are needed in the middle of the night.
- Give him 25–35 minutes from the breast he last fed on or most of his bottle feed, change his nappy and re-swaddle him.
- **Then dim the lights and, with no talking or eye contact, give him 20–25 minutes on the second breast or the remainder of the bottle feed.**
- **This should take no longer than one hour.**

**In the night**

- During the second week it is important that breast-fed babies are not allowed to go too long in the night between feeds.
- A baby weighing less than 3.2kg (7lb) at birth should be woken around 2.30am for a feed, and a baby weighing 3.2–3.6kg (7–8lb) should be woken no later than 3.30am.

- A formula-fed baby who weighs more than 3.6kg (8lb) and has fed well during the day may be able to go slightly longer, but not any longer than five hours.
- If you are in doubt as to how long to allow your baby to sleep between feeds in the night, please seek advice from your paediatrician or health visitor.

## Advancing to the two- to four-week routine

The following signs will help you decide whether you can advance on to the two- to four-week routine:

- Your baby should weigh over 3.2kg (7lb), have regained his birth weight and show signs of gaining approximately 30g (1oz) a day in weight.
- He is sleeping well at nap times and more often than not you have to wake him from his naps for him to be fed.
- He is feeding more efficiently and often emptying a breast within 25–30 minutes.
- He is showing signs of being more alert and managing to stay awake easily for an hour and a half at a time.

## Routine for a breast-feeding baby at two to four weeks

| **Feed Times** | **Nap times between 7am and 7pm** |
|---|---|
| 7am | 8.30/9am–10am |
| 10am | 11.30am/12 noon–2pm |
| 2pm | 4pm–5pm |
| 5pm | |
| 6.15pm | |
| 10.30pm | **Maximum daily sleep:** 5 hours |

Expressing times: 6.45am, 10.30am and 9.45pm

**7am**

- **Baby should be awake, nappy changed and feeding no later than 7am.**
- He needs 20–25 minutes on the full breast, then 10–15 minutes on the second breast after you have expressed approximately 60–90ml (2–3oz).
- If he fed at 5am or 6am, offer 20–25 minutes from the second breast after expressing 90ml (3oz).
- **Do not feed after 7.45am, as it will put baby off his next feed.** He can stay awake for up to two hours.

**8am**

- Try to have some cereal, toast and a drink yourself no later than 8am.

**8.45am**

- Baby should start to get a bit sleepy by this time. Even if he does not show the signs, he will be getting tired, so take him to his room now. Check his nappy and draw sheet and close the curtains.

**9am**

- Before he is asleep or before he goes into a deep sleep, settle baby in his cot, fully swaddled (see page 22), in the dark with the door shut, no later than 9am. **He needs a sleep of no longer than one and a half hours**.
- Wash and sterilise bottles and expressing equipment.

**9.45am**

- Open the curtains and unswaddle baby so that he can wake up naturally.
- Prepare things for top-and-tailing and dressing.

**10am**

- **Baby must be fully awake now, regardless of how long he slept.**
- He should be given 20–25 minutes from the breast he last fed

on while you drink a large glass of water.

- Wash and dress baby, remembering to cream all his creases.

**10.30am**

- Express 60ml (2oz) from the second breast, then offer baby 10–15 minutes. **Do not feed him after 11.15am, as it will put him off his next feed.**
- Lay him on his playmat so that he can have a good kick before he gets too tired.

**11.30am**

- If baby was very alert and awake during the previous two hours, he may start to get tired by 11.30am and would need to be in bed by 11.45am.

**11.45am**

- Regardless of what he has done earlier, he should now be taken to his room.
- Check the draw sheet and change his nappy.
- Close the curtains and **settle baby once he is drowsy, fully swaddled and in the dark with the door shut, no later than 12 noon.**

**11.30am/12 noon–2pm**

- Baby needs a nap of no longer than two and a half hours from the time he went down.
- If he slept one and a half hours earlier, only allow him two hours this nap time.
- **If he wakes up after 45 minutes check the swaddle, but do not talk to him or turn the lights on.**
- Allow 20 minutes for him to resettle himself; if he's still unsettled, offer him half his 2pm feed and try to settle him back to sleep until 2pm.

**12 noon**

- Wash and sterilise expressing equipment, then you should have lunch and rest before the next feed.

**2pm**

- **Baby must be awake and feeding no later than 2pm, regardless of how long he has slept.**
- Open the curtains, unswaddle him and allow him to wake naturally. Change his nappy.
- Give 20–25 minutes from the breast he last fed on. If he is still hungry offer 10–15 minutes from the other breast while you drink a large glass of water.
- **Do not feed after 3.15pm as it will put him off his next feed.**
- **It is very important that he is fully awake now until 4pm, so he goes down well at 7pm;** if he was very alert in the morning he may be more sleepy now. Do not put too many clothes on him, as extra warmth will make him drowsy.
- Lay him on his playmat and encourage him to have a good kick.

**4pm**

- Change baby's nappy. This is a good time to take him for a walk to ensure that he sleeps well, and is refreshed for his bath and next feed.
- **Baby should not sleep after 5pm if you want him to go down well at 7pm.**

**5pm**

- **Baby must be fully awake and feeding no later than 5pm.**
- Give him a good 20 minutes on the breast he last fed on.
- It is very important that he waits for the other breast until after his bath.

**5.45pm**

- If baby has been very wakeful during the day or didn't nap well between 4pm and 5pm, he may need to start his bath early.
- Allow him a good kick without his nappy while preparing things needed for his bath and bedtime.

**6pm**

- Baby must start his bath no later than 6pm, and be massaged and dressed by 6.15pm.

**6.15pm**

- **Baby must be feeding no later than 6.15pm; this should be done in the nursery with dim lights and no talking or eye contact.**
- If he did not empty the first breast at 5pm, allow 5–10 minutes before putting him on the full breast and give him a good 20–25 minutes on it.
- **It is very important that baby is in bed two hours from when he last awoke.**

**7pm**

- **When he becomes drowsy settle him, fully swaddled and in the dark, with the door shut, no later than 7pm.**
- If he doesn't settle within 10–15 minutes, offer him 10 minutes from the fullest breast. Do this in the dark with no talking or eye contact.

**8pm**

- It is very important that you have a really good meal and a rest before the next feed or expressing.

**9.45pm**

- If you have chosen to replace the 10.30pm breast-feed with a bottle of either breast or formula milk, then express from both breasts now.

**10/10.30pm**

- Turn up the lights fully and unswaddle baby so that he can wake up naturally. Allow at least 10 minutes before feeding to ensure he is fully awake, so that he can feed well. Baby should be fully awake and feeding by 10.30pm.
- Lay out things for the nappy change, plus a spare draw sheet, muslin and swaddle blanket in case they are needed in the middle of the night.

- Give him 20 minutes from the breast he last fed on or most of his bottle-feed, change his nappy and reswaddle him.
- Then dim the lights and with no talking or eye contact give him 20 minutes on the second breast or the remainder of the bottle-feed. This feed should take no longer than one hour.

**In the night**
- If baby wakes before 4am, give him a full feed.
- If he wakes between 4am and 5am, give him one breast, then the second at 7am after expressing.
- If he wakes at 6am, give him one breast, then the second at 7.30am after expressing.
- Make sure that you keep the lights dim and avoid eye contact or talking. Only change his nappy if absolutely necessary.

## Changes to be made during the two- to four-week routine

### Sleep

By three or four weeks your baby should start to show signs of being more wakeful and for longer periods. Ensure that you encourage the wakefulness during the day so that his night-time sleep is not affected. If possible, try to continue to put him in the nursery in the dark with the door shut for all his daytime sleeps, except the 4pm one. If school runs with older children prevent this, try at least to put him down for his lunchtime nap in his nursery in the dark. Between 7pm and 10pm, he should always be put down in the nursery and in the dark, with the door shut. If you choose to transfer him to your bedroom for the 10.30pm feed and the rest of the night, use the same settling procedure as you do in his nursery. By four weeks the morning nap should be no more than one hour, to ensure that he sleeps well at lunchtime.

Gradually, aim to keep him awake longer in the morning, until he is going down for his sleep at 9am. If you find that he is going to sleep at 8.30am and waking up between 9.15am and

9.30am, which has an adverse effect on the rest of the day, top-and-tailing him around 8.20am is usually enough to revive him sufficiently to last until 9am. If school runs prevent you from doing this and he is awake from 9.15am, you could try allowing him a short catnap of 10 minutes around 10.45am–11am. This means he would go down for his lunchtime nap somewhere between 12.15–12.30pm, avoiding the much earlier time of 11.15am if he had been awake since 9.15am. The afternoon nap should be no more than one hour in total; this nap is sometimes broken into a couple of catnaps between 4pm and 5pm.

By five weeks he should be half-swaddled (under the arms) for the 9am and the late-afternoon naps. Around four weeks it becomes more obvious when the baby comes into his light sleep: normally every 45 minutes, although it can be every 30 minutes with some babies. If a feed is not due, most babies, given the opportunity, settle themselves back to sleep. Rushing too quickly to your baby and assisting him back to sleep by rocking, patting or using the dummy could result in a long-term sleep association problem. This means that in the night when your baby comes into his light sleep, you could end up getting up several times to help him back to sleep, long after the time he no longer needs night feeds.

### Feeding

Most babies go through a growth spurt around the third week. When your baby goes through a growth spurt, reduce the amount you express at 6.45am by 30ml (1oz) and by the end of the fourth week reduce the 10.30am expressing by 30ml (1oz). This will ensure that your baby immediately receives the extra milk he needs. If you have not been expressing, you will need to allow your baby to feed more often on the breast, and for longer periods, in order for him to get the amounts he needs. During this time, try to get extra rest so that your baby's increased feeding demands do not have the opposite effect on you, causing you to become so exhausted that your milk supply decreases even further. If you do not wish to lose his sleeping routine, you could try using the plan on page 213, which increases the milk supply without losing the sleep routine. Once your milk supply has increased, you can then go back to following the routine suitable for your baby's age.

If you are breast-feeding and have decided to give one bottle-feed a day, this is a good age to introduce it. If you leave it any later than this age, it is very possible that your baby will refuse a bottle altogether, which can cause enormous problems later on, particularly if you are going back to work. It is advisable to express somewhere between 9.30pm and 10pm, totally emptying both breasts to keep your milk supply up. You will obviously not be able to express and feed your baby at 10.30pm, so whoever gives the baby his 10.30pm feed will need to follow the advice in my routines. You should get to bed early! The expressed milk can either be used for the 10.30pm feed, or frozen and used on the occasions when you need to leave your baby with a babysitter. Introducing a bottle of either expressed milk or formula at 10.30pm also allows the father to get involved and enables the mother to get to bed earlier, giving her the much-needed extra sleep that all mums need during the early weeks. If you wish to breast-feed for longer than six weeks, avoid giving formula at any other feeds, unless advised by your health visitor or paediatrician.

Bottle-fed babies should have their 7am, 10.30am and 10.30pm feeds increased first during growth spurts. Some bottle-fed babies are ready to go from using a newborn teat to a slow-flow teat.

Once your baby reaches four weeks he will probably show signs of being happy to go slightly longer between feeds, and you should be able to move him on to the four- to six-week feeding routine, provided he is regularly gaining between 180–240g (6–8oz) each week. Breast-fed babies who are not gaining sufficient weight should remain on the two- to four-week routine until their weight gain improves. Low weight gain in breast-fed babies is usually caused by a low milk supply or poor positioning at the breast, the two usually going hand in hand. It would be worthwhile following the plan for increasing your milk supply on page 213. I would also advise that you arrange a home visit from a breast-feeding counsellor to check that you are positioning your baby on the breast correctly.

If your baby is formula-fed and not gaining sufficient weight, try moving him from the newborn teat with one hole to the slow-flow teat with two holes. Always discuss any concerns you have regarding your baby's low weight gain with your health visitor or paediatrician.

If you find your baby is still waking around 2am then again at 5am, I would suggest that you wake him promptly at 10pm, give him most of his feed and keep him awake for longer than the recommended one hour. At 11.15pm his nappy should be changed and the lights dimmed in his nursery while you give him a small top-up feed. By giving him a split feed and having him awake slightly longer at this time, he will more than likely sleep well past 3am, provided he is not getting out of his covers (see page 150). In a short while this should improve and you can slowly move the feed forward to 10.30pm by five minutes each night.

## Routine for a breast-feeding baby at four to six weeks

| **Feed Times** | **Nap times between 7am and 7pm** |
|---|---|
| 7am | 9am–10am |
| 10.30am | 11.30am/12 noon–2/2.30pm |
| 2/2.30pm | 4.15pm/5pm |
| 5pm | |
| 6.15pm | |
| 10.30pm | **Maximum daily sleep:** 4½ hours |

Expressing times: 6.45am, 10.30am and 9.45pm

**7am**

- **Baby should be awake, nappy changed and feeding no later than 7am.**
- If he fed at 3am or 4am he needs 20–25 minutes on the full

breast. If he's still hungry offer 10–15 minutes from the second breast after you have expressed 60–90ml (2–3oz).
- If he fed at 5am or 6am offer 20–25 minutes from the second breast after expressing 60–90ml (2–3oz).
- **Do not feed after 7.45am, as it will put baby off his next feed.** He can stay awake for up to two hours.

**8am**
- You should try to have some cereal, toast and a drink no later than 8am.

**8.45am**
- Baby should start to get a bit sleepy by this time. **Even if he does not show the signs, he will be getting tired, so take him to his room now.**
- Check his nappy and draw sheet and close the curtains.

**9am**
- **When he is drowsy, settle baby, fully or half-swaddled and in the dark with the door shut, no later than 9am.**
- He needs a sleep of no longer than one hour.
- Wash and sterilise bottles and expressing equipment.

**9.45am**
- Open the curtains and unswaddle baby so that he can wake up naturally.
- Prepare things for top-and-tailing and dressing.

**10am**
- **Baby must be fully awake now, regardless of how long he slept.**
- Wash and dress him, remembering to cream all his creases and dry skin.

**10.30am**
- Baby should be given 20–25 minutes from the breast he last fed on.

- Lay him on his playmat so that he can have a good kick while you express 30ml (1oz) from the second breast. Then offer him 10–15 minutes.
- **Do not feed after 11.30am, as it will put him off his next feed.**

**11.30am**

- If baby was very alert and awake during the previous two hours, he may start to get tired by 11.30am and would need to be in bed by 11.45am.

**11.45am**

- Regardless of what he has done earlier, he should now be taken to his room.
- Check the draw sheet and change his nappy.
- Close the curtains and **when he is drowsy settle him, fully swaddled and in the dark with the door shut, no later than 12 noon.**

**11.30am/12 noon–2/2.30pm**

- Baby needs a nap of no longer than two and a half hours from the time he went down.
- **If he wakes up after 45 minutes, check the swaddle, but do not talk to him or turn the lights on.**
- **Allow 20 minutes for him to resettle himself;** if he's still unsettled, offer him half his 2pm feed.
- Try to settle him back to sleep until 2.30pm.

**12 noon**

- Wash and sterilise expressing equipment, then make sure you have some lunch yourself and a well-earned rest before the next feed.

**2.20pm**

- **Baby must be awake and feeding no later than 2.30pm, regardless of how long he has slept.**
- Open the curtains, unswaddle him and allow him to wake naturally. Change his nappy.

- Give 20–25 minutes from the breast he last fed on, then offer him 10–15 minutes from the other breast while you drink a large glass of water.
- **Do not feed after 3.15pm as it will put him off his next feed.**
- **It is very important that he is fully awake now until 4.15pm, so he goes down well at 7pm;** if he was very alert in the morning he may be more sleepy now. Do not put too many clothes on him, as extra warmth may make him drowsy.
- Lay him on his playmat and encourage him to have a good kick.

**4.15pm**

- Change baby's nappy. This is a good time to take him for a walk to ensure that he sleeps well in his pram, and is refreshed for his bath and next feed. He may start to cut right back on this nap.
- **Baby should not sleep after 5pm if you want him to go down well at 7pm.**

**5pm**

- **Baby must be fully awake and feeding no later than 5pm.**
- Give him a good 20 minutes on the breast he last fed on.
- **It is very important that he waits for the other breast until after his bath.**

**5.45pm**

- **If he has been very wakeful during the day, or didn't nap well between 4.15pm and 5pm, he may need to start his bath early.**
- Allow him a good kick without his nappy while preparing things needed for his bath and bedtime.

**6pm**

- He should start his bath no later than 6pm, and be massaged and dressed by 6.15pm.

**6.15pm**

- **He must be feeding no later than 6.15pm.**
- **This should be done in the nursery with dim lights and no talking or eye contact.**
- If he did not empty the first breast at 5pm, allow 5–10 minutes before putting him on the full breast.
- Give him a good 20–25 minutes on the full breast while you drink a large glass of water.
- **It is very important that he is in bed two hours from when he last awoke.**

**7pm**

- **Settle baby, fully or half-swaddled (under the arms) and in the dark with the door shut, no later than 7pm.**

**8pm**

- **It is very important for you to have a really good meal and a rest before feeding or expressing at 10/10.30pm.**

**9.45pm**

- If you have chosen to replace the 10.30pm breast-feed with a bottle of either breast or formula milk, then express from both breasts now.

**10–10.30pm**

- Turn up the lights fully and unswaddle baby so that he can wake up naturally. Allow at least 10 minutes before feeding to ensure that he is fully awake, so that he can feed well. Baby should be fully awake and feeding by 10.30pm.
- Lay out things for the nappy change, plus a spare draw sheet, muslin and swaddle blanket in case they are needed in the middle of the night.
- Give him 20 minutes from the first breast or most of his bottle-feed, change his nappy and reswaddle him.
- **Dim the lights and, with no talking or eye contact, give him 20 minutes on the second breast or the remainder of the bottle-feed.**

- **This feed should take no longer than one hour.**

**In the night**
- If he wakes up before 4am, give him a full feed.
- If he wakes between 4am and 5am give one breast, then the second at 7.30am after expressing.
- If he wakes up at 6am give him one breast, then the second at 7.30am after expressing.
- Always avoid eye contact and talking, and keep the lights low. Don't change his nappy unless absolutely necessary.

## Changes to be made during the four- to six-week routine

### Sleep

His daily nap time between 7am and 7pm should be reduced to a strict four and a half hours: the morning nap should be no more than one hour, the afternoon nap no more than 30 minutes between 4.15pm and 5pm.

If your baby is very sleepy during the day and not managing to stay awake for the suggested times, check Chapter 4 to see if this could become a real problem.

It is very important that by the end of six weeks you start to get your baby used to being half-swaddled (under the arms) at the 9am and the 7pm sleeps. Cot death rates peak between two and four months and overheating is considered to play a major factor in cot death.

It should now take less time to settle your baby to sleep. The cuddling time should gradually be reduced and now is a good time to get him used to going down when he is more awake. Often, a lullaby light which plays a tune and casts images on the ceiling for 10 minutes or so will help a baby to settle himself.

Your baby should start to sleep a longer stretch in the night around now, provided he is getting most of his daily milk intake between 6–7am and 11pm. A good indicator of this will be his weight gain; he should regularly be gaining between

180–240g (6–8oz) each week. He would also need to be staying awake for near to two hours at his social time.

Once he has done this stretch several nights in a row, try not to feed him if he suddenly goes back to waking earlier again. The hours after the 10.30pm feed are sometimes referred to as the 'core night method' (see page 207). On waking at this time he should initially be left for a few minutes to settle himself back to sleep. If that doesn't work, then other methods apart from feeding should be used to settle him. I would try settling him with some cool boiled water or a cuddle; others recommend a dummy. Attention should be kept to the minimum while reassuring the baby that you are there. This teaches the baby one of the most important sleep skills: how to go back to sleep after surfacing from a non-REM sleep. Obviously, if he refuses to settle you would need to feed him. This method could also be used to encourage an older baby, who has got into the habit of waking at the same time in the night, to sleep longer.

Before embarking on this method, the following points should be read carefully to make sure that your baby really is capable of going for a longer spell in the night:

- These methods should never be used with a very small baby or a baby who is not gaining weight.
- The above methods should only be used if your baby is regularly gaining 180–240g (6–8oz) each week, and if you are sure that his last feed is substantial enough to help him sleep for the longer stretch in the night.
- The main sign that a baby is ready to cut down on a night feed is regular weight gain and the reluctance to feed, or take less, at the 7am feed.

The aim of this method is gradually to increase the length of time your baby can go from his last feed and not to eliminate the night feed in one go. The core night method can be used if, over three or four nights, a baby has shown signs that he is capable of sleeping for a longer stretch.

## Feeding

If your baby is feeding between 3am and 4am and you have to wake him up at 7am every morning, very gradually, and by a small amount, cut back the amount of milk he is taking in the night. This will have the knock-on effect of him drinking more during the day and less in the night, and eventually he will drop the middle-of-the-night feed altogether. It is important not to cut back too much or too fast as the baby could then start to wake up hungry long before 7am, which would defeat the whole purpose of getting him to sleep through to 7am from 11pm.

Increase the day feeds, not the night feeds. Cut back on the first expressing of the day by a further 30ml (1oz) and by the end of six weeks cut out the 10.30am expressing completely. Most babies are happy to wait longer after the 7am feed, so gradually keep pushing the 10am feed forward until 10.30am. The exception to this would be a baby who is getting to nearer 5am and having a top-up at 7.30am.

It is unlikely that he would get through to 10.30am on having only a top-up feed at 7.30am, therefore continue to feed him at 10am until he is feeding between 6am and 7am.

Most babies go through a second growth spurt at six weeks, and want to spend longer on the breast at some feeds. Bottle-fed babies should have the 7am, the 10.30am and the 6.15pm feeds increased first during growth spurts. If, during this growth spurt, your baby's lunchtime nap becomes unsettled, it would be worthwhile giving him a small top-up prior to him going down for his nap. Once he has done a week of uninterrupted midday naps, gradually cut back on the top-up until you have eliminated it altogether.

If your baby is still waking twice in the night refer to page 127 for advice on splitting the 10.30pm feed.

# Routine for a breast-feeding baby at six to eight weeks

| **Feed Times** | **Nap times between 7am and 7pm** |
| --- | --- |
| 7am | 9am–9.45am |
| 10.45am | 11.45am/12 noon–2/2.30pm |
| 2/2.30pm | 4.30pm–5pm |
| 6.15pm | |
| 10.30pm | **Maximum daily sleep:** 4 hours |

Expressing times: 6.45am and 9.45pm

**7am**

- **Baby should be awake, nappy changed and feeding no later than 7am.**
- If he fed at 4am or 5am, offer him 20–25 minutes on the full breast. If he's still hungry offer 10–15 minutes from the second breast after you have expressed 30–60ml (1–2oz).
- If he fed at 6am offer him 20–25 minutes from the second breast after you have expressed 30–60ml (1–2oz).
- **Do not feed after 7.45am, as it will put him off his next feed.** He can stay awake for up to two hours.

**8am**

- Don't forget to have your own breakfast and a drink by 8am.
- Wash and dress baby, remembering to cream all his creases and dry skin.

**8.50am**

- Check his nappy and draw sheet, and close the curtains.

**9am**

- **Settle the drowsy baby, half-swaddled and in the dark with the door shut, no later than 9am.**
- He needs a sleep of no longer than 45 minutes.
- Wash and sterilise bottles and expressing equipment.

**9.45am**

- Open the curtains and unswaddle baby so that he can wake up naturally.

**10am**

- **Baby must be fully awake now, regardless of how long he slept.**
- If he had a full feed at 7am he should last until 10.45am for his next feed. If he fed earlier followed by a top-up at 7.30am, he may need to start this feed slightly earlier.
- Encourage him to have a good kick under his playgym.

**10.45am**

- He should be given 20–25 minutes from the breast he last fed on, then offered 10–15 minutes from the second breast while you have a large glass of water.
- **Do not feed after 11.30am, as it will put him off his next feed.**

**11.30am**

- If baby was very alert and awake during the previous two hours, he may start to get tired by 11.30am and would need to be in bed by 11.45am.

**11.45am**

- Regardless of what he has done earlier, he should now be taken to his room.
- Check the draw sheet and change his nappy.
- Close the curtains and **settle baby, half- or fully swaddled and in the dark with the door shut, no later than 12 noon.**

**11.45am/12 noon–2/2.30pm**

- Baby needs a nap of no longer than two and a half hours from the time he went down.

**12 noon**

- Wash and sterilise expressing equipment, then you should have lunch and a rest before the next feed.

**2.30pm**

- **Baby must be awake and feeding no later than 2.30pm, regardless of how long he has slept.**
- Open the curtains, unswaddle him and allow him to wake naturally. Change his nappy.
- Give 20–25 minutes from the breast he last fed on, then offer him 10–15 minutes from the other breast while you drink a large glass of water.
- **Do not feed after 3.15pm as it will put him off his next feed.**
- **It is very important that he is fully awake now until 4.30pm, so he goes down well at 7pm.**
- If he was very alert in the morning he may be more sleepy now. Do not put too many clothes on him, as extra warmth will make him drowsy.
- Lay him on his playmat and encourage him to have a good kick.

**4.15pm**

- Change his nappy, and offer him a drink of cool boiled water or well-diluted juice no later than 4.30pm. (If, once your baby reaches eight weeks, he refuses water, try him with water with a hint of peach juice.)
- This is a good time to take him for a walk to ensure that he sleeps well, and is refreshed for his bath and next feed.

**5pm**

- **Baby must be fully awake now if you want him to go down well at 7pm.**
- Give him 20 minutes on the breast he last fed on. It is important that he waits until after his bath for the other breast.

**5.30pm**

- Allow him a good kick without his nappy while preparing things needed for his bath and bedtime.

**5.45pm**

- He must start his bath no later than 5.45pm, and be massaged and dressed by 6.15pm.

**6.15pm**

- **He must be feeding no later than 6.15pm and this should be done in the nursery with dim lights and no talking or eye contact.**
- If he fed at 5pm, allow him a further 10–15 minutes to empty that breast completely, before putting him on the second breast.
- If he did not feed at 5pm, he should start on the breast he last fed on. Give him 20 minutes on each breast while you drink a large glass of water.
- **It is very important that he is in bed two hours from when he last woke up.**

**7pm**

- **Settle baby, half-swaddled and in the dark with the door shut, no later than 7pm.**

**8pm**

- **It is very important for you to have a really good meal and a rest before the next feed or expressing.**

**9.45pm**

- If you have chosen to replace the 10.30pm breast-feed with a bottle of either breast or formula milk, then express from both breasts now.

**10/10.30pm**

- Turn on the lights fully and unswaddle baby so that he can wake up naturally. Allow at least 10 minutes before feeding to ensure that he is fully awake, so that he can feed well. Baby should be fully awake and feeding by 10.30pm.
- Lay out things for the nappy change, plus a spare draw sheet, muslin and swaddle blanket in case they are needed in the middle of the night.
- Give him 20 minutes from the first breast or most of his bottle-feed, change his nappy and re-swaddle him.

- **Dim the lights and, with no talking or eye contact, give him 20 minutes on the second breast or the remainder of the bottle feed.**
- **This feed should take no longer than one hour.**

**In the night**

- If he is feeding well before 4am and losing interest in his 7am feed, it would be wise to try settling him with some cool boiled water. If he even takes an ounce or two before going on the breast, it should have the knock-on effect of him feeding better at 7am. The aim is to get him to take all his daily requirements between 7am and 11pm. If he is gaining 180–240g (6–8oz) of weight each week, it is important that he is encouraged to cut down and eventually drop the night feed.
- If he wakes between 4am and 5am, give one breast, then the second at 7am after expressing.
- If he wakes up at 6am, give him one breast, then the second at 7.30am after expressing.
- As before, keep the lights low and any stimulation to a minimum. No nappy change unless absolutely necessary.

## Changes to be made during the six- to eight-week routine

### Sleep

Most babies who weigh over 4kg (9lb) should be sleeping longer in the night now, provided they are getting most of their daily nutritional needs between 6–7am and 11pm. They should also be sleeping no more than four hours between 7am and 7pm. Once he has lasted longer for several nights in a row, try not to feed your baby before that time again. The morning nap should be no more than 45 minutes, the lunchtime nap should be between two and two and a half hours, no longer, and the afternoon nap should be no more than 30 minutes. He may catnap on and off during this nap; some babies cut out this nap altogether. Do not allow him to cut out this nap if he is not managing to stay awake until 7pm. If you want him to sleep until 7am, it is important that he goes to sleep nearer 7pm. If, for some reason, the lunchtime nap went wrong (see page 227), he may need slightly more sleep after the 2pm feed. Some babies will have a catnap after the 2pm feed – at around 3pm of about 15 minutes – then a further catnap around 4.30–5pm.

He should now be half-swaddled at the 9am and 7pm sleeps, and at 12 noon and from 11pm to 7am by the end of eight weeks. Some babies may start to wake up earlier in the night again once they are out of the swaddle; try to settle without feeding or fully swaddling.

### Feeding

If your baby goes back to waking up earlier again, wait 10 minutes or so before going to him. If he will not settle himself back to sleep, try settling him with some water or a cuddle. If still unsettled then feed him.

Keep increasing day feeds, not night feeds. Most babies are happy to wait longer after the 7am feed, so keep pushing this feed forward until he is feeding at 10.45am. However, if your baby is still feeding at 5–6am with a top-up at 7–7.30am he may not manage to go longer and would need to have at least half of his next feed at 10am. Most babies go through a second growth spurt at six weeks. Cut back on the first expressing of the day by a further 30ml (1oz) and by the end of eight weeks cut out the 6.45am expressing so your baby gets the extra milk he needs. He may also need to spend longer on the breast at some feeds during growth spurts.

Bottle-fed babies should have the 7am, 10.45am and 6.15pm feeds increased first during growth spurts. The 10.30pm feed should only be increased if all the other feeds have been increased, and he is not going a longer spell in the night. Try not to give more than 180ml (6oz) at this feed. Some babies will need to move to a medium-flow teat with three holes at this stage.

# Routine for a breast-feeding baby at eight to twelve weeks

| **Feed Times** | **Nap times between 7am and 7pm** |
|---|---|
| 7am | 9am–9.45am |
| 10.45/11am | 12 noon–2/2.15pm |
| 2/2.15pm | 4.45pm–5pm |
| 5pm | |
| 6.15pm | |
| 10.30pm | **Maximum daily sleep:** 3½ hours |
| Expressing time: 9.45pm | |

**7am**

- **Baby should be awake, nappy changed and feeding no later than 7am.**
- He should be given 20 minutes from the first breast, then offered 10–15 minutes from the second breast.
- **Do not feed after 7.45am, as it will put baby off his next feed.**
- He can stay awake for up to two hours.

**8am**

- Try to have some cereal, toast and a drink no later than 8am.
- Wash and dress baby, remembering to cream all his creases and dry skin.

**8.50am**

- Check his nappy and draw sheet, and close the curtains.

**9am**

- **Settle the drowsy baby, half-swaddled and in the dark with the door shut, no later than 9am.**
- He needs a sleep of no longer than 45 minutes.
- Wash and sterilise bottles and expressing equipment.

**9.45am**

- Open the curtains and unswaddle baby so that he can wake up naturally.

**10am**

- Baby must be fully awake now, regardless of how long he slept.
- Encourage him to have a good kick under his playgym.

**10.45/11am**

- Baby should be given 20 minutes from the breast he last fed on, then offered 10–15 minutes from the second breast while you have a large glass of water.
- **Do not feed after 11.30am, as it will put him off his next feed.**

**11.45am**

- Regardless of what he has done earlier, he should now be taken to his room.
- Check the draw sheet and change his nappy.
- Close the curtains and **settle baby, half-swaddled and in the dark with the door shut, no later than 12 noon.**

**12 noon–2/2.15pm**

- Baby needs a nap of no longer than two and a quarter hours from the time he went down.
- Wash and sterilise bottles and expressing equipment.

**2/2.15pm**

- **Baby must be awake two and a quarter hours from the time he went down, regardless of how long he has slept, and he must be feeding no later than 2.30pm.**
- Open the curtains, unswaddle him and allow him to wake naturally. Change his nappy.
- Give 20 minutes from the breast he last fed on, then offer him 10–15 minutes from the other breast while you drink a large glass of water.

- **Do not feed after 3.15pm as it will put him off his next feed.**
- **It is very important that he is fully awake now until 4.45pm, so he goes down well at 7pm.**

**4.15pm**

- Change his nappy, and offer him a drink of cool boiled water or well-diluted juice no later than 4.30pm.
- He may have a short nap between 4.45pm and 5pm.

**5pm**

- **Baby must be fully awake if you want him to sleep at 7pm.**
- If he is very hungry offer him 10–15 minutes on the breast he last fed on, otherwise try to get him to wait until after his bath for a full feed. By 12 weeks he should be happy to wait until after his bath for his feed.

**5.30pm**

- Allow him a good kick without his nappy while preparing things needed for his bath and bedtime.

**5.45pm**

- He must start his bath no later than 5.45pm, and be massaged and dressed by 6.15pm.

**6.15pm**

- **He must be feeding no later than 6.15pm and this should be done in the nursery with dim lights and no talking or eye contact.**
- He should be given 20 minutes on each breast while you drink a large glass of water.
- **It is very important that he is in bed two hours from when he last awoke.**

**7pm**

- **Settle the drowsy baby, half-swaddled and in the dark with the door shut, no later than 7pm.**

**8pm**

- **It is very important for you to have a really good meal and a rest before the next feed or expressing.**

**9.45pm**

- If you have chosen to replace the 10.30pm breast-feed with a bottle of either breast or formula milk, then express from both breasts now.

**10/10.30pm**

- Turn on the lights fully and unswaddle baby so that he can wake up naturally. Allow at least 10 minutes before feeding to ensure that he is fully awake, so that he can feed well. Baby should be feeding by 10.30pm.
- Lay out things for the nappy change, plus a spare draw sheet, muslin and swaddle blanket in case they are needed in the middle of the night.
- Give him 20 minutes on the first breast or most of his bottle-feed, change his nappy and re-swaddle him.
- **Dim the lights and, with no talking or eye contact, give him 20 minutes on the second breast or the remainder of the bottle-feed.**
- **This feed should take no longer than one hour.**

**In the night**

- If your baby is feeding before 5am, feeding well and losing interest in his 7am feed, it would be wise to try settling him with some cool boiled water. Remember, the aim is to get him to take all his daily requirements between 7am and 11pm. As long as he is gaining 180g (6oz) a week, he can be encouraged to go through to 5am without a milk feed.
- If he wakes up at 5am give him the first breast and, if needed, 5–10 minutes on the second breast.
- If he wakes up at 6am, give the first breast, then the second at 7.30am.
- Avoid night-time stimulation; only change his nappy if necessary.

# Changes to be made during the eight- to twelve-week routine

## Sleep

Most babies who weigh nearer 5.4kg (12lb) in weight should manage to go through the night from the 10.30pm feed at this age, provided they are taking all their daily nutritional needs between 7am and 11pm. They should also be sleeping no more than three and a half hours between 7am and 7pm. A totally breast-fed baby may still be waking up once in the night, hopefully nearer 5am or 6am.

Cut back your baby's daily nap time by a further 30 minutes, to a total of three hours. The morning nap should be no more than 45 minutes, but if he is not sleeping so well at lunchtime, it can be cut back to 30 minutes. The lunchtime nap should be no more than two and a quarter hours. It is around this stage that the lunchtime nap can sometimes go wrong. The baby comes into a light sleep usually 30–45 minutes after he has gone to sleep. Some babies will wake up fully and it is important that they learn how to settle themselves back to sleep if the wrong sleep associations are to be avoided. For more details on this problem refer to Chapter 8.

Most babies have cut back their late-afternoon nap, but if this is not so, do not allow more than 15 minutes, unless for some reason the lunchtime nap has gone wrong, and then it would be slightly longer but not run past 5pm. All babies should only be half-swaddled and sleeping in their big cots; particular attention should be paid when tucking the baby in the cot.

One reason many babies of this age still wake up is because they move around the cot and get their arms and legs caught between the spars. If this is happening with your baby, I would advise that you purchase one of the very light summer-weight sleeping bags from the company named at the back of the book. They are so lightweight that you can still use a sheet and one blanket to tuck them in, without the worry of overheating. (See pages 3–6 for further details on cots and bedding.)

### Feeding

He should be well established on five feeds a day now and sleeping all or most of the night. If he is totally breast-fed and has started waking up earlier in the morning, it may be worth trying a top-up from a bottle of either expressed or formula milk after you feed him at 10.30pm. If he is sleeping regularly to 7am, gradually bring the 10.30pm feed forward by five minutes every three nights until he is feeding at 10pm. As long as he continues to sleep through to 7am and takes a full feed, then you can keep taking the 10.45am feed back until he is feeding at 11am.

If your baby isn't sleeping through the night, you could go back to splitting the 6.15pm feed and give him 10–15 minutes at 5pm. Cut the 5pm feed out once he is sleeping through regularly for 2–3 weeks.

If you are considering introducing a further bottle-feed, the best time to introduce it is at the 11am feed. Gradually reduce the time of the feed by two or three minutes each day and top up with formula. By the end of the first week, if your baby is taking a bottle-feed of 150–180ml (5–6oz), you should be able to drop the breast-feed easily without the risk of serious engorgement (see page 61 for further advice). Bottle-fed babies should continue to have their 7am, 11am and 6.15pm feeds increased first during the next growth spurt at around nine weeks. Increase the bottle-feed to suit your baby's needs.

## Routine for a baby at three to four months

| **Feed Times** | **Nap times between 7am and 7pm** |
|---|---|
| 7am | 9am–9.45am |
| 11am | 12 noon–2/2.15pm |
| 2.15/2.30pm | |
| 6.15pm | |
| 10.30pm | **Maximum daily sleep:** 3 hours |

Expressing time: 9.45pm

**7am**

- **Baby should be awake, nappy changed and feeding no later than 7am.**
- He should feed from both breasts or take a full bottle-feed and then should stay awake for two hours.

**8am**

- He should be encouraged to have a good kick on his playmat or enjoy other activities for 20–30 minutes.
- Wash and dress baby, remembering to cream all his creases and dry skin.

**9am**

- **Settle the drowsy baby, half-swaddled and in the dark with the door shut, no later than 9am.** He needs a sleep of no longer than 45 minutes.
- Wash and sterilise bottles and expressing equipment.

**9.45am**

- Open the curtains and unswaddle him so that he can wake up naturally.

**10am**

- **Baby must be fully awake now, regardless of how long he slept.**
- Encourage him to have a good kick under his playgym.

**11am**

- He should be given a feed from both breasts or a full bottle-feed.
- Do not feed after 11.30am as it will put him off his next feed.

**11.50am**

- Check the draw sheet and change his nappy.
- Close the curtains and **settle the drowsy baby, half-swaddled and in the dark with the door shut, no later than 12 noon.**

**12 noon–2/2.15pm**

- Baby needs a nap of no longer than two and a quarter hours from the time he went down. Wash and sterilise bottles and expressing equipment.

**2/2.15pm**

- **Baby must be awake two and a quarter hours from the time he was put to bed, regardless of how long he has slept, and he must be feeding no later than 2.30pm.**
- Open the curtains, unswaddle him and allow him to wake naturally, then change his nappy.
- He needs a feed from both breasts or a bottle-feed.
- **Do not feed him after 3.15pm as it will put him off his next feed.**
- If he has slept well at both naps he should manage to get through the rest of the afternoon without a further sleep.

**4.15pm**

- **Change his nappy and offer him a drink of cool boiled water or well-diluted juice no later than 4.30pm.**

**5.30pm**

- Put him on the changing mat on the floor without his nappy, so that he can have a good kick while your prepare his bath.

**5.45pm**

- Baby must start his bath no later than 5.45pm, and be massaged and dressed no later than 6.15pm.

**6.15pm**

- **He must be feeding no later than 6.15pm.**
- He should feed from both breasts or have a full formula-feed.
- Dim the lights and sit him in his chair for 10 minutes while you tidy up.

**7pm**

- **Settle the drowsy baby, half-swaddled and in the dark with the door shut, no later than 7pm.**

**9.45pm**

- If you have chosen to replace the 10.30pm breast-feed with a bottle of either breast or formula milk, you can express both breasts now.

**10.30pm**

- Turn the lights on low and wake him enough to feed. He should be fully awake and feeding by 10.30pm.
- Give him most of his breast-feed or formula-feed, change his nappy and half swaddle him.
- **Dim the lights and, with no talking or eye contact give him the remainder of his feed. If he does not want the remainder do not force it, as he should start to cut back on this feed now.**
- This feed should take no longer than 30 minutes.

## Changes to be made during the three- to four-month routine

### Sleep

If you have structured the milk feeds and nap times according to the routine, your baby should manage to sleep through the night from his last feed to nearer 6–7am. If he shows signs of starting to wake up earlier it would be advisable to assume that it may be hunger and increase his 10.30pm feed and, if need be, go back to having him awake longer at that feed (see page 127). You should also ensure that his maximum daily sleep between 7am and 7pm totals no more than three hours. Most babies will cut right back on their late-afternoon sleep and some days may manage to get through the afternoon without the nap, but may need to go to bed 5–10 minutes earlier on those days.

If, for some reason, your baby has slept for less than two hours at lunchtime he should certainly be encouraged to have a short nap of no longer than 30 minutes between 4 and 5pm, otherwise he may become so overtired at bedtime that he doesn't settle to sleep easily.

The time your baby is awake at the 10.30pm feed should be gradually reduced to 30 minutes, provided he is sleeping through regularly to 7am. This feed should be a very quiet feed, and treated as a middle-of-the-night feed. If he is still waking up between 5 and 6am it would be advisable to try and keep him awake for a least an hour at the last feed.

Even if he is not getting out of his half-swaddle, I would suggest that now is a good time to get him used to a 100 per cent cotton very lightweight sleeping bag. He would still need to be tucked in firmly, with one sheet, and perhaps one blanket, depending on the room temperature; therefore it is important that you purchase a 0.5tog bag to avoid the risk of overheating.

### Feeding

If your baby is formula-fed and is taking 1050–1200ml (35–40oz) of formula between 7am and 11pm, he should not really need to feed in the night. However, some very big babies who weigh over 6.8kg (15lb) at this stage may still need to feed between 5–6am, followed by a top-up at 7–7.30am until he reaches six months and is weaned. Current guidelines are that babies are not weaned before six months. If you are concerned that your baby is showing all the signs of needing to be weaned, it is important that you discuss this with your health visitor or paediatrician.

It is better to keep feeding in the night for a slightly longer time than take the risk of weaning your baby before he is ready. A totally breast-fed baby may also need to feed around 5–6am as he may not be getting enough to eat at the last feed. Regardless of whether they are breast- or bottle-fed, a good indicator of whether your baby is ready to drop the night feed is how he takes his top-up at 7–7.30am. If he takes it greedily he is probably genuinely hungry at 5–6am. If he fusses and frets and refuses the top-up, I would assume the early wake-up was more habit than hunger and try to settle him back with some cool boiled water or a cuddle.

If your baby continues to sleep through to 7am once his waking time at 10.30pm has been reduced to 30 minutes, plus he is cutting back on his 7am feed, start reducing the amount he is drinking at 10.30pm. Only continue with this if he is sleeping well until 7am. However, I would not advise dropping this feed altogether until he reaches six months and solids have been established. If you abandon the 10.30pm feed before solids are introduced and he goes through a growth spurt, you may find that you have to go back to feeding him in the middle of the night again.

If your baby is totally breast-fed and is over 6.3kg (14lb) in weight, you may find that during growth spurts you have to go back to feeding him in the middle of the night anyway, until solids are introduced.

## Routine for a baby at four to six months

| **Feed Times** | **Nap times between 7am and 7pm** |
|---|---|
| 7am | 9am–9.45am |
| 11am | 12 noon–2/2.15 pm |
| 2.15/2.30pm | |
| 6pm | |
| 10.30pm | **Maximum daily sleep:** 3 hours |
| Expressing time: 9.45pm | |

**7am**

- **Baby should be awake, nappy changed and feeding no later than 7am.**
- He should feed from both breasts or have a full bottle-feed and should then stay awake for two hours.

**8am**

- He should be encouraged to have a good kick on his playmat or enjoy other activities for 20–30 minutes.
- Wash and dress baby, remembering to cream all his creases and dry skin.

**9am**

- **Settle the drowsy baby, half-swaddled and in the dark with the door shut, no later than 9am.** He needs a sleep of no longer than 45 minutes.
- Wash and sterilise bottles and expressing equipment.

**9.45am**

- Open the curtains and unswaddle him so that he can wake up naturally.

**10am**

- **Baby must be fully awake now, regardless of how long he slept.**
- Encourage him to have a good kick under his playgym or take him on an outing.

**11am**

- He should be given a full breast-feed or a full bottle-feed before being offered solids, if you have been advised to wean early (see page 165).
- Encourage him to sit in his chair while you clear away the lunch things.

**11.50am**

- Check the draw sheet and change his nappy.
- Close the curtains and **settle the drowsy baby, half-swaddled and in the dark with the door shut, no later than 12 noon.**
- **He will need a nap now of no longer than two and a quarter hours from the time he went down.**

**2/2.15pm**

- Open the curtains, unswaddle him and allow him to wake naturally. Change his nappy.
- He needs a feed from both breasts or a full bottle-feed.
- **Do not feed him after 3.15pm as it will put him off his next feed.**
- If he has slept well at both naps he should manage to get through the rest of the afternoon without a further sleep.

**4.15pm**

- Change baby's nappy and offer him a drink of cool boiled water or well-diluted juice no later than 4.30pm.
- If he did not sleep so well at lunchtime, he may need a short nap now.

**5pm**

- He should be happy to go to after the bath for his feed, but if he is showing signs of hunger, then offer a small feed now.
- Put him on the changing mat on the floor without his nappy, so that he can have a good kick while your prepare his bath.

**5.30pm**

- He must start his bath around now, and be massaged and dressed no later than 6pm.

**6pm**

- **He should start his feed between 6pm and 6.15pm, depending on how tired he is.**
- He should feed from both breasts or have a full bottle-feed.

**7pm**

- **Settle the drowsy baby, half-swaddled or in his sleeping bag and in the dark with the door shut, no later than 7pm.**

**9.45pm**

- If you have chosen to replace the 10.30pm breast-feed with a bottle of either breast or formula milk, you can express from both breasts now.

**10.30pm**

- Turn the lights on low and wake him enough to feed. Baby should be fully awake and feeding by 10.30pm.
- Give him most of his breast- or bottle-feed, change his nappy and half swaddle him.
- **Dim the lights and with no talking or eye contact, give him the remainder of the feed. If he does not want the remainder do not force it, as he should start to cut back on this feed now.**
- This feed should take no longer than 30 minutes.

# Changes to be made during the four- to six-month routine

## Sleep

Between four and six months your baby should manage to sleep from his last feed at 10.30pm until 6/7am, provided he is taking 4–5 full milk feeds a day, and not sleeping more than 3 hours between 7am and 7pm. If you have not already introduced a sleeping bag it would be advisable to do so at this stage. To leave it any later you may risk the problem of him being unhappy when he is eventually put into one.

Until he is able to crawl and manoeuvre himself around the cot, he needs to be tucked in firmly. In very hot weather he can be put into a 0.5tog bag with just a nappy on and tucked in with a very thin cotton sheet.

If he is not sleeping the full two hours at lunchtime, cut back his morning nap to 20–30 minutes, and bring the 11am feed forward to 10.30am, then top him up at midday with some milk, before he goes down for his lunchtime nap.

## Feeding

I would recommend that you still continue to feed him at 10.30pm until solids are established. The current guidelines are that solids should now be introduced at six months, rather than at four months as previously recommended. As your baby will continue to go through growth spurts between four and six months, his nutritional needs will still need to be met. In my experience, this can rarely be done on four milk feeds a day. If you decide to drop the 10.30pm feed and he starts to wake earlier and not settle back to sleep quickly, then you should assume that it is hunger and feed him. It would be then worth considering re-introducing the 10.30pm feed until solids are established. If you find that he refuses a 10pm feed, but wakes up at 5am hungry, then you should feed him and settle him back to sleep until 7am, then offer him a top-up feed before 8am. If this happens, you may then have to feed him earlier, between 10am and 10.30am, but I would suggest that you offer him a further top-up before he goes down for his lunchtime nap, to ensure that he does sleep well.

During growth spurts you may find that your baby is not content on five feeds a day, and you may have to offer a split feed as mentioned above in the morning, and also re-introduce the 5pm feeds again.

If your baby becomes very discontent between feeds, despite your offering him extra milk, and you think that he is showing signs of needing to be weaned (for more detail see page 166), then it is important that you discuss this with your health visitor or doctor. If they advise that your baby needs to be weaned before the recommended six months, then it is important that you introduce solids very carefully. Solids should only be seen as tasters at this stage and given in addition to milk, not to replace milk feeds.

To ensure that this does not happen always make sure that your baby takes all of his milk feed first. Start off with a small amount of baby rice mixed with either breast milk or formula milk after the 11am feed. Once he is taking this you can then transfer the rice to after the 6pm feed in the evening, then start to introduce some of the first weaning foods recommended on page 172 after the 11am feed.

If you find that your baby is too tired to take all of his milk at 6pm followed by the solids, then give him two-thirds of the milk at 5.15pm, followed by the solids, followed by the remainder of his milk feed at 6.45pm.

Once solids are introduced at this feed, and as they increase, he should automatically cut back on his last feed at 10.30pm. Once he down to taking only a very short breast-feed or just a couple of ounces of formula at 10.30pm, and continuing to sleep well through to 7am, you should be able to drop the 10.30pm feed without risking that he will wake earlier in the morning.

## Routine for a baby at six to nine months

| **Feed Times** | **Nap times between 7am and 7pm** |
|---|---|
| 7am | 9am–9.30/45am |
| 11.45am | 12.30pm–2.30pm |
| 2.30pm | |
| 5pm | |
| 6.30pm | **Maximum daily sleep:** 3 hours |

**7am**

- **Baby should be awake, nappy changed and feeding no later than 7am.**
- He should feed from both breasts or have a full bottle-feed, followed by breakfast cereal mixed with either expressed milk or formula and fruit.
- He should stay awake for two hours.

**8am**

- He should be encouraged to have a good kick on his playmat or enjoy other activities for 20–30 minutes.
- Wash and dress baby, remembering to cream all his creases and dry skin.

**9am**

- **Settle the drowsy baby, in his sleeping bag (see page 150) in the dark with the door shut between 9am and 9.30am.**
- He needs a sleep of 30–45 minutes.

**9.30/9.45am**

- Open the curtains and undo his sleeping bag so that he can wake up naturally.

**10am**

- **Baby must be fully awake now, regardless of how long he slept.**
- Encourage him to have a good kick under his playgym or take him on an outing.

**11.45am**

- He should be given most of his solids before being offered a drink of water or well-diluted juice from a beaker, then alternate between solids and a drink.
- Encourage him to sit in his chair while you clear away the lunch things.

**12.20pm**

- Check the draw sheet and change his nappy.
- **Close the curtains and settle the drowsy baby, in his sleeping bag in the dark with the door shut, no later than 12.30pm.**

**12.30pm–2.30pm**

- **He will need a nap now of no longer than two hours from the time he went down.**
- If he slept the full 45 minutes earlier, he may need less sleep at this nap.

**2.30pm**

- **Baby must be awake and feeding no later than 2.30pm, regardless of how long he has slept.**

- Open the curtains, unswaddle him and allow him to wake up naturally. Change his nappy.
- He needs a feed from both breasts or a full bottle-feed.
- **Do not feed him after 3.15pm as it will put him off his next feed.**

**4.15pm**
- Change baby's nappy and offer him a drink of cool boiled water or well-diluted juice no later than 4.30pm.

**5pm**
- He should be given most of his solids before being offered a small drink of water from a beaker. It is important that he still has a good milk feed at bedtime, so keep this drink to a minimum.

**6pm**
- He must start his bath no later than 6pm, and be massaged and dressed no later than 6.30pm.

**6.30pm**
- **Baby must be feeding no later than 6.30pm.**
- He should feed from both breasts or have 210ml (7oz) of formula-feed.
- Dim the lights and sit him in his chair for 10 minutes while you tidy up.

**7pm**
- **Settle the drowsy baby in his cot and in the dark with the door shut, no later than 7pm.**

## Changes to be made during the six- to nine-month routine

### Sleep

Once your baby is established on three meals a day, he should manage to sleep from around 7pm to 7am. If you have followed the most recent guidelines on weaning and started weaning your baby on to solids at six months, he will probably need a small feed at 10.30pm until he is nearer seven months. If you were advised to wean him before six months and solids were well established when he reached six months, you should be able to drop the 10.30pm feed sooner.

Once he reaches six months, and provided he is sleeping soundly to 7am most mornings, you should aim to keep pushing the 9am nap forward to 9.30am. This will encourage him to go down for his lunchtime nap nearer to 12.30pm. This is important once solids are established and he is having three proper meals a day, with lunch coming around 11.45–noon.

Some babies are happy to sleep later in the morning once they are established on three solid meals a day. If your baby sleeps until nearer 8am, he will not need a morning nap, but may not manage to get through until 12.30pm for his lunchtime nap; therefore, he may need to have lunch around 11.30am so he can go down at 12.15pm for his lunchtime nap.

Between six and nine months he will also start to roll on to his front and prefer to sleep on his tummy. When this happens, it would be advisable to remove the sheet and blanket so as to avoid him getting into a tangle. In the winter months, the lightweight sleeping bag will need to be replaced with a warmer one to make up for the loss of blankets.

### Feeding

If you have waited until six months to introduce solids, it is important that you work through the foods groups fairly quickly (see page 174). Introduce baby rice after the 11am feed, and then every couple of days introduce a new food, and keep increasing the amounts. Once your baby is taking a reasonable amount of solids at lunchtime and teatime, you can introduce solids at breakfast. By seven months your baby must be having protein foods at lunchtime, as he will have used up all the iron stored in his body when he was born.

If you were advised to wean your baby earlier than normally recommended, you should be able to introduce protein foods as soon as he reaches six months, as his digestive system will be used to digesting different types of foods by this stage.

It is also important that you introduce your baby to a beaker at lunchtime between the ages of six and seven months, and that you start to use the tier system of feeding at lunchtime. Once your baby is only taking a couple of ounces of milk at lunchtime, replace it with a drink of water or well-diluted juice from a beaker. It is important that this is done once your baby is eating protein at lunchtime. Once the lunchtime milk is dropped, he may need to increase the 2.30pm feed. However, if you notice that he is cutting back too much on his last feed, continue to keep this feed smaller.

Between six and seven months, solids should be transferred and changed to a proper tea at 5pm, with only a small drink of water from a beaker, if you have not already done this. He would then have a full milk feed around 6.30pm.

By nine months, if your baby is formula-fed, he should be drinking all of his water, diluted juice and most of his milk feeds from a beaker.

## Routine for a baby at nine to twelve months

| **Feed Times** | **Nap times between 7am and 7pm** |
|---|---|
| 7am | 9.15/9.30am–10am |
| 11.45am | 12.30pm–2.30pm |
| 2.30pm | |
| 5pm | |
| 6.30pm | **Maximum daily sleep 3 hours** |

**7am**

- **Baby should be awake, nappy changed and feeding no later than 7am.**

- He should feed from both breasts or have a drink of formula from a beaker, followed by breakfast cereal mixed with either expressed milk or formula and fruit.
- He should stay awake for two to two and a half hours.

**8am**
- He should be encouraged to have a good kick on his playmat or enjoy other activities for 20–30 minutes.
- Wash and dress baby, remembering to cream all his creases and dry skin.

**9.15/9.30am**
- **Settle the drowsy baby in the dark with the door shut.**
- He needs a sleep of 30–45 minutes.

**9.30–9.45am**
- Open the curtains so that he can waken up naturally.

**10am**
- **Baby must be fully awake now, regardless of how long he slept.**
- Encourage him to have a good kick under his playgym or take him on an outing.

**11.45am**
- He should be given most of his solids before being offered a drink of water or well-diluted juice from a beaker, then alternate between solids and a drink.
- Encourage him to sit in his chair while you clear away the lunch things.

**12.20pm**
- Check the draw sheet and change his nappy.
- Close the curtains and **settle baby in the dark with the door shut, no later than 12.30pm. He will need a nap now of no longer than two hours from the time he went down.**

- If he slept the full 45 minutes earlier, he may need less sleep at this nap.

**2.30pm**

- **Baby must be awake and feeding no later than 2.30pm, regardless of how long he has slept.**
- Open the curtains, and allow him to wake up naturally. Change his nappy.
- **He needs a breast-feed or formula milk, water or well-diluted juice from a beaker.**
- **Do not feed him after 3.15pm as it will put him off his supper.**

**4.15pm**

- Change baby's nappy and offer him a drink of cool boiled water or well-diluted juice no later than 4.30pm.

**5pm**

- He should be given most of his solids before being offered a small drink of water or milk from a beaker. It is important that he still has a good milk feed at bedtime, so keep this drink to a minimum.

**6pm**

- He must start his bath no later than 6pm, and be massaged and dressed no later than 6.30pm.

**6.30pm**

- **He must be feeding no later than 6.30pm.**
- He should feed from both breasts or have a full bottle-feed; the amount will eventually be reduced to 150–180ml (5–6oz) when a beaker is introduced at one year.
- Dim the lights and sit him in his chair for 10 minutes while you tidy up.

**7pm**

- Settle him in his cot, in the dark with the door shut, no later than 7pm.

# Changes to be made during the nine- to twelve-month routine

## Sleep

The majority of babies cut right back on their daily sleep at this stage. If you notice that your baby is starting to wake earlier in the morning, it is important that you cut back on his total daily sleep.

The first nap to cut back on is the morning one. If he is having 45 minutes, then try cutting it back to 30 minutes. If he has been having only 30 minutes, then cut it back to 10–15 minutes. Some babies may also cut right back their lunchtime nap to one and a half hours, which can lead to them to becoming very tired and irritable in the late afternoon. If this happens to your baby, try cutting out the morning nap altogether to see if it improves his lunchtime sleep. You may have to bring lunch forward slightly if he can't make it through to 12.30pm for his nap.

Your baby may also start to pull himself up in the cot, but become very upset when he can't get himself back down. If this happens, it would be advisable to encourage him to practise laying himself down when you put him down for his naps. Until he is able to manoeuvre himself up and down, you would need to go in and help him settle back down. It is important that this is done with the least fuss and talking.

## Feeding

If your baby starts to cut back on his last milk feed, reduce, or cut out altogether, the 2.30pm feed. Many babies cut out the 2.30pm feed by one year. As long as he is getting a minimum of 350ml (12oz) of milk a day, inclusive of milk used in cereal and cooking, he will be getting enough.

He should be well established on three meals a day, and should also be able to feed himself some of the time. At nine months, a formula-fed baby should be taking all of his breakfast milk and 2.30pm feed from a beaker.

By the age of one year, he should be drinking all his milk and other fluids from a beaker.

# Introducing solid food 7

## Weaning your baby

The latest Department of Health (DoH) guidelines were published in 2003 and were prompted by recommendations from the World Health Organisation. They advise exclusive breast-feeding for the first six months of a baby's life, i.e. no solids or infant formula. The previous DoH advice was to wean between four and six months and not to give solids to any baby before 17 weeks. This is because it takes up to four months for the lining of a baby's gut to develop and for the kidneys to mature enough to cope with the waste products from solid food. If solids are introduced before a baby has the complete set of enzymes required to digest food properly, his digestive system could become damaged. Many experts blame the rapid increase in allergies over the last 20 years on babies being weaned before their digestive system is ready to cope.

During the writing of the latest edition of this book, I have spoken to many dietitians and paediatricians as well as to hundreds of mothers via my website. It is clear that there is some controversy surrounding these recommendations. Certainly, there are health professionals who feel that it is not weaning between four and six months which threatens a baby's health, but the kind of food the baby is given. It is also clear that there are many babies who cannot manage on milk alone for the full six months. I urge you to discuss any and all of your concerns with your health visitor or GP and to follow their advice accordingly.

The golden rules are: that your baby should not be given

food before 17 weeks; nor should weaning begin before neuromuscular co-ordination has developed sufficiently, so that the baby can control his head and neck while sitting upright supported in a chair to be fed. He should also be able to swallow food easily, by moving it from the front of his mouth to the back.

If you follow the weaning plan in this book and introduce the recommended foods in the order suggested, you can be confident that you are not putting your baby at risk of food allergies. Babies rely on the introduction of iron-containing foods at six months, as their bodies' iron stores, with which they are born, become depleted at this age. Iron is essential for healthy red blood cells that transport oxygen around the body. Children who do not take in sufficient amounts of iron are at risk of developing iron-deficiency anaemia which causes tiredness, irritability and an overall lack of energy and enthusiasm. Up to a quarter of 18-month-old children in the UK show signs of iron deficiency anaemia, so if a breast-fed baby is weaned at six months, it is important that iron-containing foods, such as breakfast cereals, broccoli, lentils and baby foods with iron are introduced swiftly. You will need to progress quickly through the food groups to include meat or vegetarian alternatives for their iron content. Babies on formula will have their iron supplemented in the milk.

I do not know your baby and cannot tell you when he is ready to wean. All babies should be watched closely for signs that they are ready for weaning, which might possibly come sooner than the current DoH recommendations. If your baby is under six months of age and showing all the signs below, it is vital you discuss things with your health visitor or GP and decide with them whether to wean early or not.

I hope the guidelines below will help you identify possible signs of being ready to wean. A baby could be ready if:

- He has been taking a full feed four or five times a day from both breasts or a 240ml (8oz) bottle of formula and has been happily going for four hours between feeds, but now gets irritable and chews his hands long before his next feed is due.

- He has been taking a full feed from both breasts, or a 240ml (8oz) formula feed, and screams for more the minute the feed finishes.
- He usually sleeps well at night and nap times but is starting to wake up earlier and earlier.
- He is chewing his hands excessively, displaying eye-to-hand co-ordination and trying to put things into his mouth.

If your baby is over four months old, has doubled his birthweight and is consistently displaying most of these signs, he could be ready to begin weaning. If the baby is under six months you should tell your health visitor or GP and decide how to proceed. If you decide to wait until the baby is six months before you introduce solids, it is important that his increased hunger is met by introducing further milk feeds. Babies who have been sleeping through the night with only a small feed at 10.30pm would need to have this feed increased. And, if they go through a further growth spurt before they reach six months, it may be that you need to introduce a further feed in the middle of the night. It is very important to understand that as your baby grows, so will his appetite. If you wish to continue exclusive breast-feeding until six months it is unreasonable to expect the baby to manage on only four milk feeds a day.

### Breast-fed babies

With babies who are being breast-fed exclusively it is more difficult to tell how much milk they are receiving. If your baby is over four months and showing most of the above signs, you will need to talk to your health visitor or GP about the choices available to you.

If he is under four months and not gaining enough weight each week, it is possible that your milk supply is getting very low in the evening. All that may be needed is extra milk. I suggest you try topping up the baby with a couple of ounces of expressed or formula milk after the 10.30pm feed. If this does not work, or if he is waking up more than once in the night, I would replace the 10pm feed altogether with a full bottle-feed, if you have not already done so. Encourage your partner to do this feed so that you can get to bed early, after expressing whatever milk you have between 9.30 and 10pm to avoid your supply dropping any further. Mothers in this situation often find that when they express they are only producing 90–120ml (3–4oz), which is much less than their baby may need at this feed. The milk expressed can, if necessary, be given at some other feed during the day, thus avoiding further complementary bottle-feeding.

This plan usually satisfies a baby's hunger, and improves his weight gain. You should never wean a baby before 17 weeks of age and, if sooner than six months, it should be done only on medical advice.

## Foods to be avoided

During the first two years of your baby's life certain foods are best used sparingly, or avoided altogether, as they may be harmful to your baby's health. The two worst culprits in this regard are sugar and salt.

### Sugar

During the first year of weaning, it is best to avoid adding sugar to any of your baby's food, as it may lead to him developing a taste for sweet things. A baby's appetite for savoury foods can be seriously affected if he is allowed lots of food containing sugar or sugar substitutes. But when buying commercial foods these ingredients can be hard to avoid. A survey by the Consumer's Association magazine, *Which?*, tested 420 baby products and reported that 40 per cent contained sugar or fruit juice or both. When choosing baby cereals or commercial foods, check the labels carefully; sugar may be listed as dextrose, fructose, glucose or sucrose. Watch out, too, for syrup or concentrated fruit juice, which are also sometimes used as sweeteners.

Too much sugar in the diet may not only cause your baby to refuse savoury food, but can lead to serious problems such as tooth decay and obesity. Because sugar converts very quickly into energy, babies and children who have too much may become hyperactive. Products such as baked beans, spaghetti hoops, cornflakes, fish fingers, jam, tomato ketchup, tinned soups and some yoghurts are just a few of the everyday foods that contain hidden sugars, so care should be taken that when your baby reaches toddlerhood he does not eat these foods in excess. It is also important to check the labels of fruit juices and squashes.

### Salt

Children under two years of age should not have salt added to their food – they get all the salt they need from natural sources such as vegetables. Adding salt to a young baby's food can be very dangerous, as it may put a strain on his immature kidneys. Research also shows that children with high salt intake may be more prone to heart disease later. When your baby reaches the important stage of joining in with family meals, it is important that you do not add salt to the food during cooking. Remove your baby's portion, then add salt for the rest of the family.

As with sugar, many processed foods and commercially prepared meals contain high levels of salt. It is important to check the labels on these foods carefully before giving them to your toddler.

## Preparing and cooking food for your baby

Making your own food not only often works out cheaper, but, more importantly, will be of great nutritional benefit for your baby. And it needn't be fiddly or time-consuming if you make up large quantities at a time and store mini meals away in the freezer. Keep sterilised feeding equipment, ice cube trays and freezerproof containers at the ready and follow the general instructions below:

- When preparing food, always ensure that all surfaces are clean and have been wiped down with an anti-bacterial cleaner. Use kitchen roll for cleaning surfaces and drying, as it is more hygienic than kitchen cloths and towels, which may carry bacteria.
- All fresh fruit and vegetables should be carefully peeled, removing the core, pips and any blemishes. They should then be rinsed thoroughly with filtered water.
- If you are advised to wean your baby early, remember that all fruit and vegetables must be cooked until your baby is six months old. This can be done by either steaming or boiling in filtered water. Do not add salt, sugar or honey.
- During the initial stages all food must be cooked until soft enough to purée to a very smooth consistency. A small amount of the cooking water may need to be added so that the mixture is similar to smooth yoghurt.
- If using a food processor, check carefully for lumps by using a spoon and pouring into another bowl. Then transfer to ice cube trays or containers for storage in the freezer.

### Sterilised feeding equipment

All feeding equipment should be sterilised for the first six months, and bottles and teats for as long as they are used. Sterilise ice cube trays or freezer containers by boiling them in a large saucepan of water for five minutes. Use a steam steriliser, if you have one, for small items such as spoons or serving bowls, and follow timings recommended in the manufacturer's handbook. Wash cooking utensils as usual in a dishwasher or rinse handwashed items with boiling water from the kettle.

### Packing food for the freezer

- Make sure cooked, puréed food is covered as quickly as possible and transfer it to the freezer as soon as it's cool enough.
- Never put warm food into a refrigerator or freezer.
- Check the temperature of your freezer on a freezer thermometer. It should read –18°C. If you don't have a freezer thermometer, they can be bought from a good hardware shop or the cookware section of a large department store.
- If using an ice cube tray, fill with puréed food, open-freeze until solid, then pop the cubes out of the tray and into a sterilised plastic box. Non-sterilised items such as plastic bags can be used from six months. Seal well and freeze.
- Label items clearly, adding the date.
- Use foods within six months.
- Never refreeze cooked food. Food can only be put back into the freezer if it was originally frozen raw then defrosted and cooked – a raw frozen chicken breast, defrosted, for example, can be frozen as a cooked casserole.

### Defrosting tips

- Defrost frozen (covered) food in the fridge overnight or leave at room temperature if you forget, transferring it to the fridge as soon as it has defrosted. Make sure it is covered at all times and stand it on a plate to catch the drips.
- Never speed up defrosting by putting food into warm or hot water.
- Always use defrosted foods within 24 hours.

### Reheating tips

- Food should be heated thoroughly to ensure that any bacteria are killed. If using jars, always transfer to a dish; never serve straight from the jar. Any food left over should be discarded, never reheated and used again.

- When batch cooking, take out a portion of food for your baby to eat now and freeze the rest. Don't be tempted to reheat the entire mixture and then freeze what is left.
- If your baby has only eaten a tiny portion it can be tempting to reheat and serve leftovers later. Please don't – babies are much more susceptible than adults to food poisoning, so get in the habit of throwing leftovers away immediately.
- Reheat foods only once.

## Early weaning

If you have been advised that your baby is ready for weaning before the recommended age of six months remember that milk is still the most important food for him. It provides him with the right balance of vitamins and minerals. Solids given before six months are classed as first tastes and fillers which should be increased very slowly over several weeks, gradually preparing your baby for three solid meals a day. By offering the milk first you will ensure that his daily milk intake does not decrease too rapidly before he reaches six months.

Studies into weaning by the University of Surrey revealed that babies fed diets with a high fruit content may be more prone to diarrhoea, which leads to slow growth. They advise that baby rice is the best first weaning food as fruit may not be so well tolerated by the under-developed gut of some babies.

Remember that as soon as your baby has teeth and has begun on any type of solid food, he will need his teeth cleaning twice a day, preferably after each meal.

### How to begin

- Introduce solids after the 11am feed. Prepare everything you need for giving the solids in advance: a baby chair, bib, spoon, bowl and a clean, fresh damp cloth.
- Start by offering your baby a teaspoonful of pure organic rice mixed to a very smooth consistency using either expressed milk, formula or cool, filtered freshly boiled water.

- Make sure the baby rice has cooled enough before feeding it to your baby. Use a shallow plastic spoon for him – never a metal one, which can be too sharp or get too hot.
- Some babies need help in learning how to feed from the spoon. By placing the spoon just far enough into his mouth, and bringing the spoon up and out against the roof of his mouth, his upper gums will take the food off, encouraging him to feed.
- Once your baby is established on baby rice at 11am and is tolerating it, give the rice after the 6pm feed instead. When he finishes the one teaspoonful and shows signs of looking for more food, the amount of solids can be increased, provided he continues to take the required amount of milk at 6pm.
- Once your baby is happily taking 1–2 teaspoonfuls of baby rice mixed with milk or water after the 6pm feed, a small amount of pear purée can be introduced after the 11am feed. With babies under six months this usually happens between the fourth and sixth day, and with babies over six months it will probably happen between the second and fourth day.
- Be guided by your baby as to when to increase the amounts. He will turn his head away and get fussy when he has had enough.
- If the baby tolerates the pear purée, transfer it to the 6pm feed. Mixing the purée with baby rice in the evening will make it more palatable and prevent your baby from getting constipated.
- Small amounts of various organic vegetables and fruit can now be introduced, one by one, after the 11am feed. To prevent your baby from developing a sweet tooth, try to give more vegetables than fruit. At this stage, avoid the stronger-tasting ones such as spinach or broccoli, but rather concentrate on root vegetables (such as carrot, sweet potato and swede). These contain natural sugars, will taste sweeter and blander, and may prove more palatable to your baby.
- With babies under six months it is important to introduce new foods in small amounts and every 3–4 days. Increasing

1–2 teaspoonfuls a week between the two meals is a good guideline. Babies over six months will probably need their meals increased by larger amounts every couple of days, and as long as you stick to the foods listed in first stage weaning you can introduce new foods closer together. Keeping a food diary will help you see how your baby reacts to each new food.

- If your baby spits a food out, it may not mean he dislikes it. Remember this is all very new to him and different foods will get a different reaction. If he positively refuses a food, however, leave it and try again in a week's time.
- Always offer milk first, as this is still the most important food at this stage in nutritional terms. While appetites do vary, in my experience the majority of babies will be drinking 840–900ml (28–30oz) of formula a day, or 4–5 full breast-feeds. Provided your baby is happy and thriving, once solids are introduced the minimum daily recommended amount of milk can be reduced to 600ml (20oz) a day.

For more comprehensive advice on weaning, including daily plans and recipes you can prepare for your baby, see *The Contented Little Baby Book of Weaning*. There are many more easy-to-prepare recipes for babies and toddlers in *The Gina Ford Baby and Toddler Cook Book*.

## First stage: six to seven months

If your baby started weaning before six months he will probably have tasted baby rice, plus a variety of different vegetables and fruits. Follow my guidelines (see page 172) for when to start baby rice and when to introduce fruit and vegetables. Once you have started weaning it is important to keep introducing a variety of the different fruits and vegetables listed below in the first-stage weaning foods. All fruit and vegetables should still be steamed or cooked in filtered water until soft, then puréed. Mix to the desired consistency with some of the cooking water, or chicken stock may be used with some vegetables.

You should avoid introducing dairy products, wheat, eggs, nuts and citrus fruit as they are the foods most likely to trigger allergies. Honey should not be introduced before one year. Meat, chicken and fish should not be introduced until the babies are capable of digesting reasonable amounts of other solids. Some nutritionists believe that protein can put a strain on the young baby's kidneys and digestive tract. I agree. All too often I have seen feeding problems occur because meat, poultry or fish have been introduced too early. Once you have worked through the first foods you can introduce protein. In the meantime, your first sources of iron can be found in lentils, broccoli and iron-rich breakfast cereals.

When beginning weaning at the age of six months you will need to progress quickly through the first-stage foods so the iron-rich meat and vegetarian products can be introduced regularly. A rough guideline would be to increase the baby rice at teatime by one teaspoonful of rice every couple of days and the savoury at lunchtime by one cube every couple of days. It is also essential to rapidly reduce your baby's milk intake to four feeds a day once solids are established.

Between six and seven months, depending on when you began weaning, your baby should be having 2–3 servings of carbohydrates daily in the form of cereal, wholemeal bread, pasta or potatoes. He should each also have three servings of vegetables or fruit each day and one serving of animal or vegetable protein.

## Foods to introduce

Pure organic baby rice, pear, apple, carrot, sweet potato, potatoes, green beans, courgettes and swede are ideal first weaning foods. Once your baby is happily taking these foods, you can introduce parsnips, mango, peaches, broccoli, avocados, barley, peas and cauliflower.

Protein should be introduced by the seventh month once solids are established: lentils, poultry, fish and meat. Check that all the bones are removed and trim off the fat and the skin. Some babies find the flavour of protein cooked on its own too strong. Try cooking chicken or meat in a casserole with familiar root vegetables, and fish in a milk sauce until your baby becomes accustomed to the different texture and taste. Cook meat with vegetables as a casserole and pulse in a food processor.

Start introducing protein at lunchtime as it is harder to digest than carbohydrate and will be digested by bedtime.

### Breakfast

A baby is ready to start having breakfast once he shows signs of hunger long before his 11am feed. This usually happens between the ages of six and seven months (and when the late feed is dropped). All cereal should be wheat- and gluten-free until the age of six months. I find that organic oatmeal cereal with a small amount of puréed fruit is a favourite with most babies.

You should still give your baby most of his milk feed first; after a couple of weeks give about two-thirds of his milk feed first, then the cereal, finishing with the remainder of the milk feed. If your baby reaches seven months and shows no sign of wanting breakfast, it would be wise to reduce his milk feed very slightly and offer a small amount of solids.

### Lunchtime

Start by replacing some of the vegetable cubes you introduced at the 11am feed with two cubes of the more simple chicken, fish, meat or pulse recipes (see *The Contented Little Baby Book of Weaning* and *The Gina Ford Baby and Toddler Cook Book*). Introduce new protein foods very slowly during the early stage. A new food every three days is about right, taking careful note of what he eats and any reactions he might have. Increase the amount by one or two cubes a day until your baby's meals consist totally of one of the protein recipes.

### Introducing a beaker

Once protein is introduced at lunchtime, the milk feed should be replaced by a drink of water or well-diluted juice from a beaker. Most babies of six months are capable of sipping and swallowing, and this should be encouraged by being consistent and always offering the lunchtime drink from a beaker. Do not worry if your baby only drinks a small amount at this meal; you will probably find that he makes up for it at his 2.30pm milk feed.

### Tea

At some point during the sixth month, the cereal and fruit given at the 6pm feed can be replaced by a proper (vegetarian) tea at 5pm. If you always make sure that your baby has a well-balanced breakfast and lunch you can be relaxed about this meal. Once breakfast and lunch are established, you can sit the baby down at 5pm and offer him a small tea. Some babies can get very fractious around this time of the day, so offer foods that are quick and easy to prepare – thick vegetable soups and vegetable bakes that have been prepared and frozen in advance are always a good standby. Pasta, or a baked potato, served with vegetables and a sauce is also nutritious and easy. A very hungry baby can also be offered a milk pudding or yoghurt.

### Daily requirements

By six months a baby who started weaning early will probably be established on two solid meals a day and heading towards a third. Getting the balance of solids right is vital, so that he continues to get the right amount of milk. Although he will have cut down on the 11am breast- or bottle-feed of milk as his intake of solids increases, he still needs a minimum of 600ml (20oz) of milk a day, divided between 4–5 feeds. Babies who started weaning at six months could still be having 4–6 milk feeds a day, which you need to reduce rapidly if solids are not to be refused.

Some babies who are still drinking large amounts of milk at six months may be resistant to the introduction of solids. If you find that your baby is fussy about taking solids you should only offer him half his milk at the 11am feed to encourage interest in the solid food. You should aim to have your baby on two meals a day within a couple of weeks of beginning solids. By the time he reaches seven months, regardless of when he began weaning, all babies should be well established on two meals a day, progressing to three meals consisting of a wide variety of foods from the different food groups.

At the end of six months a typical day's menu may look something like this:

| | |
|---|---|
| **7–7.30am** | **Breakfast** |
| | Breast-feed or 210–240ml (7–8oz) of formula milk. |
| | Oat cereal mixed with milk and fruit *or* |
| | Toast with fruit spread. |
| **11.30am** | **Lunch** |
| | Chicken casserole *or* |
| | Vegetable and lentil shepherd's pie *or* |
| | Steamed fish with creamed vegetables. |
| | **Mid-afternoon** |
| | Breast-feed or 150–210ml (5–7oz) of formula milk. |
| **5pm** | **Tea** |
| | Baked potato with creamed vegetables *or* |
| | Pasta with red pepper sauce. |
| | Milk pudding or yoghurt. |
| | Small drink of water from a beaker. |
| **6.30pm** | Breast-feed or 180–240ml (6–8oz) of formula milk. |

Once a baby is established on three good solid meals a day, plus three or four full milk feeds, he should manage to go nearer to 12 hours without a feed. If your baby is not cutting down on his 10pm feed once solids are introduced it may be that he is not getting the right quantities of solids for his age or weight, or too small a feed at 6.30pm. Keep a diary of all food and milk consumed over a period of four days to help pinpoint why he is not cutting that last feed.

By the end of six months your baby will probably be ready to sit in a high chair for his meals. Always ensure that he is properly strapped in and never left unattended.

## Second stage: seven to nine months

During the second stage of weaning, the amount of milk your baby drinks will gradually reduce as his intake of solids increases. It is, however, important that he still receives a minimum of 500–600ml (17–20oz) a day of breast or formula milk. This is usually divided between three milk feeds and milk used in food and cooking, as sauces are introduced. At this stage of weaning you should be aiming at establishing three good solid meals a day, so that by the time your baby reaches nine months of age he is getting most of his nourishment from solids. During this time it is important to keep introducing a wide variety of foods from the different food groups (carbohydrate, protein, dairy, fruit and vegetables) so that your baby's nutritional needs are met.

Most babies are ready to accept stronger-tasting foods at this age. They also take pleasure from different textures, colours and presentation. Foods should be mashed or 'pulsed' and kept separate to avoid mixing everything up. Fruit need not be cooked; it can be grated or mashed. It is also around this age that your baby will begin to put food in his mouth. Raw soft fruit, lightly cooked vegetables and toast can be used as finger foods. They will be sucked and squeezed more than eaten at this stage, but allowing your baby the opportunity to feed himself encourages good feeding habits later on. Once your baby is having finger foods, always wash his hands before a meal and never leave him alone while he is eating.

Between eight and nine months your baby may show signs of wanting to use his spoon. To encourage this, use two spoons when you feed him. Load one for him to try and get the food into his mouth. You use the other for actually getting the food in! You can help his co-ordination by holding his wrist gently and guiding the spoon into his mouth.

### Foods to introduce

Dairy products, pasta and wheat can be introduced at this stage. Full-fat cow's milk can be used in cooking, but should not be given as a drink until one year. Small amounts of unsalted butter can also be used in cooking. Egg yolks can be introduced, but must be hard-boiled. Cheese should be full fat, pasteurised and grated, and preferably organic. Olive oil can be used when cooking casseroles.

Canned fish such as tuna may also be included, but choose fish in vegetable oil, as fish canned in brine has a higher salt content. A greater variety of vegetables can also be introduced such as coloured peppers, Brussels sprouts, pumpkin, cabbage and spinach. Tomatoes and well-diluted unsweetened fruit juices can be included if there is not a history of allergies. All these foods should be introduced gradually and careful notes made of any reactions.

Once your baby is used to taking food from a spoon, vegetables can be mashed rather than puréed. Once he is happy taking mashed food you can start to introduce small amounts of finger food. Vegetables should be cooked until soft then offered in cube-sized pieces or steamed and then mixed to the right consistence. Once your baby is managing softly cooked pieces of vegetables and soft pieces of raw fruit, you can try him with toast or a low-sugar rusk. By nine months, if your baby has several teeth he should be able to manage some chopped raw vegetables. Dried fruit can also be given now but it should be washed first and soaked overnight.

### Breakfast

Sugar-free, unrefined wheat cereals can now be introduced; choose those fortified with iron and B vitamins. You may want to delay introducing these if you have a family history of allergies – check with your health visitor, GP or a dietitian. Try adding a little mashed or grated fruit if your baby refuses them. Try to alternate the cereals between oat-based and wheat-based, even if your baby shows a preference for one over the other. You can encourage your baby with finger foods by offering him a little buttered toast at this stage. Once your baby is finger feeding, you can offer a selection of fruits and yoghurts along with lightly buttered toast.

Most babies are still desperate for their milk first thing in the morning, so allow him two-thirds of his milk first. Once he is nearer nine months of age he will most likely show signs of not being hungry for milk and this is the time to try offering breakfast milk from a beaker.

### Lunch

If your baby is eating a proper breakfast you will be able to push lunch to somewhere between 11.45am and 12 noon. However, should he be eating only a small amount of breakfast, lunch will need to come slightly earlier. Likewise, babies who are having only a very short nap in the morning may also need to have lunch earlier. It's important to remember that overtired, hungry babies will not feed as well, so take your timing of lunch from your baby.

During this stage of weaning you will have established protein at lunchtime. Whenever possible, try to buy organic chicken and meat which is free from additives and growth stimulators. Pork, bacon and processed hams should not be introduced as they have a high salt content. You should still continue to cook without additional salt or sugar, although a small amount of herbs can be introduced at around nine months of age.

Once protein is well established, your baby's milk feed should be replaced at lunchtime by a drink of cool, boiled water or well-diluted juice from a beaker. You might find that he only drinks a small amount from the beaker and looks for an increase of milk on the 2.30pm feed or an increase of cool, boiled water later in the day.

If you are introducing your baby to a vegetarian diet, it is important to seek expert advice on getting the right balance of amino acids. Vegetables are incomplete sources of amino acids when cooked separately and need to be combined correctly to provide your baby with a complete source of protein.

If your baby is still hungry after his main meal, offer a piece of cheese, a breadstick, chopped fruit or yoghurt.

### Tea

Once your baby is finger feeding, tea can include a selection of mini-sandwiches, rice cakes with spread and breadsticks. Some babies get very tired and fussy by teatime. If your baby does not eat much, try offering some rice pudding or a yoghurt. A small drink of water from a beaker can be offered after the tea. Do not allow too large a drink at this time as it will put him off his last milk feed. His bedtime milk feed is still important at this stage. If he starts cutting back too much on this feed, check you are not overfeeding him on solids or giving him too much to drink.

### Daily requirements

At this second stage of weaning it is important that you work towards establishing your baby on three proper meals a day. They should include three servings of carbohydrates, such as cereals, bread and pasta, plus at least three servings of vegetables and fruit, and one serving of puréed meat, fish or pulses. By six months a baby has used up all the store of iron he was born with. As their requirements between six and 12 months are particularly high, it is important that their diet provides the right amount of iron. To help iron absorption in cereals and meat, always serve with fruit or vegetables, and avoid giving milk to drink with protein as it reduces the iron content by 50 per cent.

Your baby still needs 500–600ml (17–20oz) of breast or formula milk a day, inclusive of milk used for mixing food. If your baby starts to reject his milk, try giving him more cheese, milk sauces and yoghurt. By the end of nine months try to encourage your baby to drink all of his breakfast milk from a beaker. Apart from his bedtime milk, all other milk feeds and drinks should ideally be from a beaker.

A very hungry baby who is taking three full milk feeds a day, plus three solid meals, may need a small drink and a piece of fruit mid-morning.

A typical day for an eight- to nine-month-old baby would look like this:

| | |
|---|---|
| **7–7.30am** | **Breakfast** |
| | Breast-feed or 210–240ml (7–8oz) of formula milk in a beaker. |
| | Mixed mashed fruit and yoghurt *or* |
| | Wheat/oat cereal with milk and mashed fruit. |
| **11.45am/** | **Lunch** |
| **12 noon** | Chicken, broccoli and pasta in a cream sauce *or* |
| | Fish cakes with cabbage and lyonnaise potatoes. |
| | Fruit and yoghurt. |
| | Drink of water or well-diluted juice from a beaker. |
| **5pm** | **Tea** |
| | Baked potato with grated cheese and apple *or* |
| | Vegetable lasagne. |
| | Drink of water or well-diluted juice from a beaker. |
| **6.30pm** | Breast-feed or 180–240ml (6–8oz) of formula milk. |

## Third stage: nine to twelve months

Between nine and 12 months your baby should be eating and enjoying all types of food, with the exception of food with a high fat, salt or sugar content. Peanuts and honey should also still be avoided. It is very important that your baby learns to chew properly at this stage. Food should be chopped or diced, although meat still needs to be pulsed or very finely chopped. By the end of his first year, he should be able to manage chopped meat. This is also a good time to introduce raw vegetables and salads. Try to include some finger foods at every meal, and if he shows an interest in holding his own spoon, do not discourage these attempts. It is important that he enjoys his meals even if a certain amount of it lands on the floor.

### Breakfast

Encourage your baby to take at least some of his breakfast milk feed from a beaker. By the end of the first year he should be drinking all of his breakfast milk from a beaker. Aim to get him to take 210ml (7oz) of milk at this meal, divided between a drink and his breakfast cereal. Scrambled egg can be offered once or twice a week as a change.

### Lunch

Lunch should consist of a selection of lightly cooked chopped vegetables, a serving of carbohydrate in the form of potato, pasta or rice served with a serving of animal or vegetable protein. Babies of this age are very active and can become quite tired and irritable by 5pm. By ensuring a well-balanced lunch, you will not need to worry if tea is more relaxed. By the end of the first year your baby's lunch can be integrated with the family lunch. Prepare the meal without salt, sugar or spices, reserve a portion for your baby, then add these for the rest of the family.

Try to ensure that his meals are attractively presented, with a variety of different-coloured vegetables and fruit. Do not overload his plate; serve up a small amount and, when he finishes that, replenish his plate. This also helps to avoid the game of throwing food on the floor, which often occurs at this stage. If your baby does start to play up with his main course, refusing to eat and throwing food around, quietly and firmly say 'no' and remove the plate. Do *not* offer him a biscuit or fromage frais half an hour later, as a pattern will soon emerge where he will refuse lunch knowing he will get something sweet if he plays up enough. A piece of fruit can be offered mid-afternoon to see him through to tea, at which time he will probably eat very well.

A drink of well-diluted, pure, unsweetened orange juice in a beaker will help the absorption of iron at this meal, but make sure your baby has most of his meal before you allow him to finish the drink.

## Tea

Many babies cut out their 2.30pm milk during this stage. If you are worried that your baby's daily milk intake is too low, try giving him things like pasta and vegetables with a milk sauce, baked potatoes with grated cheese, cheesy vegetable bake or mini-quiches at teatime. Teatime is usually the meal when I would give small helpings of milk pudding or fromage frais, which are also alternatives if milk is being rejected. Try regularly to include some finger foods at teatime.

The bedtime bottle should be discouraged after one year, so during this stage get your baby gradually used to less milk at bedtime. This can be done by offering him a small drink of milk with his teatime meal, then a drink of 150–180ml (5–6oz) of milk from a beaker at bedtime.

## Daily requirements

By one year it is important that large volumes of milk are discouraged; no more than 600ml (20oz), inclusive of milk used in food, should be allowed. After one year your baby needs a minimum of 350ml (12oz) a day. This is usually divided between two or three drinks and is inclusive of milk used in cooking or on cereals.

Full-fat, pasteurised cow's milk can be given to drink after one year. If your baby refuses cow's milk, try gradually diluting his formula with it until he is happy to take full cow's milk. If possible try to give your baby organic cow's milk as it is higher in Omega 3 fatty acids than non-organic milk. Omega 3 fatty acids are essential for maintaining a healthy heart, supple and flexible joints, healthy growth and strong bones and teeth so it is important to make sure your baby is getting enough of them through his food.

Encourage three well-balanced meals a day and avoid snacks of biscuits, cakes and crisps. Every day aim for your baby to have 3–4 servings of carbohydrate, 3–4 servings of fruit and vegetables, and one portion of animal protein or two of vegetable protein.

By one year your baby's menu should look something like this:

| | |
|---|---|
| **7–7.30am** | **Breakfast** |
| | Breast-feed or a drink of formula milk in a beaker. |
| | Wholewheat or oat cereal with milk and fruit *or* |
| | Baby muesli with milk and fruit *or* |
| | Scrambled egg on toast *or* |
| | Yoghurt and chopped fruit. |
| **12 noon** | **Lunch** |
| | Cold, creamed chicken with apple and celery salad *or* |
| | Beef meatballs in tomato sauce with cabbage and mashed potatoes *or* |
| | Tuna burgers and mixed vegetables *or* |
| | Irish stew with parsley dumplings. |
| | Drink of water or well-diluted juice from a beaker. |
| | Yoghurt and fresh fruit. |
| | **Mid-afternoon** |
| | Drink of milk, water or well-diluted juice from a beaker. |
| **5pm** | **Tea** |
| | Thick soup and savoury sandwiches *or* |
| | Vegetarian pizza with green salad *or* |
| | Chickpea and spinach croquettes with a home-made tomato sauce *or* |
| | Lentil and vegetable lasagne. |
| | Small drink of milk, water or well-diluted juice from a beaker. |
| **6.30pm** | Breast-feed or 180ml (6oz) of formula milk from a beaker. |

# Your questions answered

**Q How will I know when my baby is ready to be weaned?**

A
- If your baby has been sleeping through and starts to wake up in the night or very early in the morning, and will not settle back to sleep.
- A bottle-fed baby would be taking in excess of 960–1140ml (32–38oz) a day, draining a 240ml (8oz) bottle each feed and looking for another feed long before it is due.
- A breast-fed baby would start to look for a feed every 2–3 hours.
- Both breast- and bottle-fed babies would start to chew on their hands a lot and be very irritable in between feeds.
- If unsure, always talk to your health visitor or paediatrician, and especially if your baby is less than six months old.

**Q What would happen if I weaned my baby before he was ready?**

A
- His digestive system could be harmed if he has not developed the complete set of enzymes required to digest solids.
- Introducing solids before he is ready could lead to allergies.
- Studies from several different countries show that persistent coughs and wheezing are more common in babies that were weaned before 17 weeks.

**Q At what milk feed should I introduce solids?**

A
- I usually start at the 11am feed as this feed will gradually be pushed to 12 noon, becoming a proper lunch once solids become established by the end of the first year.
- Milk is still the most important source of food. By giving solids after this feed you can be sure that your baby will have at least half of his daily milk intake before noon.

- Solids offered at the 2.30pm feed seem to put babies off the very important 6pm feed.
- If a very hungry baby has no adverse reaction to the baby rice within three days, I would then transfer the rice to after the 6pm feed.

**Q Which is the best food to introduce?**

A
- I find pure organic baby rice is the food that satisfies most babies' hunger the best. If this is tolerated I would then introduce some organic puréed pear.
- Once these two foods are established, it is best to concentrate on introducing a variety of vegetables from the How to Begin stage on page 173.
- In a survey carried out by the University of Surrey it was found that babies weaned on fruit were less likely to thrive than babies weaned on baby rice. They advise that all babies should start weaning on baby rice.

**Q How will I know how much solid food to give my baby?**

A
- For the first six months, milk is still the most important part of your baby's diet. It will provide him with the right balance of vitamins and minerals, so once solids are introduced he will need a minimum of 600ml (20oz) a day. During the first weeks of weaning, if you always offer the milk feed first, then the solids, you can be sure he will take exactly the amount of solids he needs. This avoids him replacing his milk too quickly with solids.
- Once you have established rice and some purées you can start at the 11am feed to give half the milk feed first, then some solids followed by more milk. This will encourage your baby to cut back slightly on his milk feed and increase his solids, preparing him for a feeding pattern of three meals a day at seven months.
- For breast-fed babies, a feed from one breast can be classed as half a milk feed.

**Q At what age do I start to cut out milk feeds altogether?**

A
- Assuming your baby was on five milk feeds when he started to wean, once he increases his solids after the 6pm feed, he should automatically cut back on his 10pm feed, then cut it out altogether. If you wean at six months, you will probably need to keep the 10.30pm feed. Once solids are established it should be easy to cut out.
- The next feed to cut out would be the 11–11.30am feed. Once your baby is having chicken or fish for lunch the milk feed should be replaced with a drink of water or well-diluted juice from a beaker.
- The 2.30pm feed often increases for a few months then, somewhere between nine and twelve months, he will lose interest in this feed, at which time it can be dropped.

**Q At what age would you introduce a drinking beaker and at which feeds?**

A
- Between the age of six and seven months is the best time.
- When you have replaced the lunchtime milk feed with water or well-diluted juice, try giving it from a beaker or a bottle with a hard spout.
- Try halfway through the meal and after every few spoonfuls of food.
- It is important to persevere. Experiment with different types of beaker until you find one with which your baby is happy.
- Once he is taking a few ounces from a beaker, gradually introduce it at other feeds.

**Q When can I introduce cow's milk?**

A
- I usually introduce a small amount of organic cow's milk in cooking from six months.
- Cow's milk should not be given as a drink until your baby is at least one year old.
- It should always be full-fat pasteurised milk, preferably organic.
- If your baby refuses cow's milk, try mixing half that

amount with formula. Once he is happy taking that, gradually increase the cow's milk until he is happy with all cow's milk.

**Q At what age can I stop puréeing my baby's food?**

A
- Once your baby has taken well to puréed food (hopefully by the end of the sixth month), you can start to mash the vegetables and fruit really well, so that there are no lumps, but it is not so smooth as the puréed food.
- Between six and nine months I gradually mash the food less and less until the babies will take food with lumps in it.
- Chicken and meat should still be pulsed until your baby is around 10 months old.

**Q When will he be able to manage finger foods?**

A
- Once your baby starts to grab at the spoon, give him one to hold.
- When he repeatedly puts it in his mouth, load up another spoon and let him try to get it into his mouth, quickly popping in any food that falls out with your spoon.
- With a little help and guidance, most babies from 12 months are capable of feeding themselves with part of their meal.
- Always supervise your baby during mealtimes. Never ever leave him alone.

**Q When can I stop sterilising?**

A
- Bottles should be sterilised until your baby is one year old.
- Dishes and spoons can stop being sterilised when your baby is six months old. They can then be put in the dishwasher, or washed thoroughly in hot soapy water, then rinsed and left to air-dry.
- After six months, the pots, cooking utensils and ice cube trays used for preparing weaning food can either be put in the dishwasher or washed in hot soapy water, rinsed and then have boiled water poured over them before being left

to air dry. If you are weaning before six months, the equipment should be sterilised.

**Q Which foods are most likely to cause allergies and what are the main symptoms?**

A
- The most common foods that cause allergies are dairy products, wheat, fish, eggs and citrus fruits.
- Symptoms include rashes, wheezing, coughing, running nose, sore bottom, diarrhoea, irritability and swelling of the eyes.
- Keeping a detailed record when you are weaning can be a big help when you are trying to establish the cause of any of the above symptoms.
- The above symptoms can also be caused by the house mite, animal fur, wool, and certain soaps and household cleaning agents.
- If in doubt, always check with your doctor to rule out any other possible causes or illness for the above symptoms.

# Common problems in the first year

# 8

I hope that the CLB routines and the advice that I give in this book will go a long way towards helping you keep problems to a minimum. However, for various reasons it is natural that problems may occur during the first year. In this chapter, I have collected together the most common problems encountered by parents during this year and I hope it will cover the majority of your concerns. Remember to consult your doctor or health visitor with any worries – even if they seem small and you fear looking like a neurotic mother. It's better that you are not beset with worries and can enjoy your baby and this precious first year together.

You can use the list of headings on the contents page (page vi) to find the problems that concern you. I have divided the information into three sections – general, feeding and sleeping problems – but many of them overlap. Sleeping and feeding are interdependent so you may find it more helpful to read this entire chapter.

## General

### Burping

It is important to follow your baby's lead regarding when to stop and wind him during feeding. If you constantly interrupt his feed to try and get his wind up, he will be more likely to get so upset and frustrated that the crying will cause more wind than the feed itself. Time and time again I watch babies being thumped endlessly on the back, the mother refusing to continue with the feed as she is convinced the baby has wind. The reality is that very few babies need to be burped more than once during a feed and once at the end.

A breast-feeding baby will pull himself off the breast when he is ready to burp. If he has not done so by the end of the first breast, you can try burping him before putting him on the second breast. Bottle-fed babies will normally drink half to three-quarters of their feed and pull themselves off to be burped. Regardless of whether you are breast-feeding or bottle-feeding, if you adopt the correct holding position as illustrated on pages 54 and 67, your baby should bring his wind up quickly and easily both during and at the end of the feed. If your baby does not bring up the wind within a few minutes it is best to leave it and try later. More often than not he will bring it up after he has been laid flat for his nappy change.

Occasionally a baby passing excessive wind from his rear end can suffer considerable discomfort and become very distressed. A breast-feeding mother should keep a close eye on her diet to see if a particular food or drink is causing the wind. Citrus fruits or drinks taken in excess can sometimes cause severe wind in some babies. The other culprits are chocolate and excessive dairy intake.

Special care should be taken to make sure that the baby is reaching the hind milk. Too much fore milk can cause explosive bowel movements and excessive passing of wind.

With a bottle-fed baby who is already feeding from the special anti-colic bottles, the cause of excessive wind is usually overfeeding. If your baby is regularly drinking 90–180ml (3–6oz) a day more than the amount advised on the packet, and constantly putting on in excess of 240g (8oz) of weight each week, cut back on a couple of his feeds (either the 2.30pm or 5pm) for a few days to see if there is any improvement. A 'sucky' baby could be offered a dummy after the smaller feeds to satisfy his sucking needs.

Sometimes a teat with a hole either too small or too large for your baby's needs could cause excessive wind. Experiment with the different sizes of teats; sometimes using a smaller hole at a couple of the feeds can help a baby who is drinking some of his feeds too quickly.

## Colic

Colic is a common problem for babies under three months. It can make life miserable for the baby and the parents, and to date there is no cure for it. There are over-the-counter medications, but most parents with a baby suffering from severe colic say that they are of little help. Although a baby can suffer from colic at any time of the day, the most common time seems to be between 6pm and midnight. Parents resort to endless feeding, rocking, patting, driving the baby round the block, most of which seem to bring little or no relief. Colic usually disappears by four months of age, but by that time the baby has often learnt all the wrong sleep associations, so the parents are no further forward.

Parents who contact me for help with their 'colicky' baby describe how the baby screams, often for hours at a time, thrashes madly and keeps bringing his legs up in pain. These babies seem to have one thing in common: they are all being fed on demand. Feeding this way all too often leads to the baby having a feed before the first one has been digested, one of the reasons that I believe may cause colic. (See also the advice on feeding bottles on page 17.)

Not one of the babies I have cared for has ever suffered from colic and I am convinced that it is because I structure their feeding and sleeping from day one. When I do go in to help an older baby who is suffering from colic it seems to disappear within 24 hours of them being put on to the routine.

Firstly, I would check that the colic was being caused by demand-feeding and not the mother's diet. Then, depending on the age, the symptoms of the baby, and how often they were feeding throughout the evening and the middle of the night, I would introduce sugar water. With a baby between one and three months of age who was feeding excessively in the night and consistently putting on more than the recommended weight gain each week, I would try to replace one of the night feeds with some sugar water. When the baby woke in the night I would give 120ml (4oz) of cool boiled water mixed with half a teaspoon of sugar to settle him. At this stage I find plain boiled water does not have the same effect. The following day I would wake the baby at 7am, regardless of how little sleep he had in the night, and then proceed with the routine throughout the day to 6.30pm. At this time I would always offer a breast-fed baby a top-up of expressed milk to ensure that he has had enough to drink. This avoids him needing to feed again in two hours, which is a common pattern of babies suffering from colic. With a bottle-fed baby I always make sure that the 2.30pm feed is smaller so that he feeds well at 6.30pm.

With an older baby of three months or more I would attempt to eliminate middle-of-the-night feeds altogether, or at least reduce the feeding to only one. In both cases it is important to ensure that the baby feeds well at 6.15pm, if necessary offering a top-up of expressed milk at this time. A low milk supply in the early evening is often the cause of a baby feeding little and often, which can lead to him not digesting feeds properly.

More often than not, the baby settled well the first night, but occasionally I worked with a baby who had developed the wrong sleep associations, as a result of the colic. With these babies I used the controlled crying method of sleep training and within 3–4 nights they were going down happily and sleeping well until the 10.30pm feed. Because they had slept well and had gone a full four hours since their last feed, they fed well and went on to last for an even longer spell in the night. Depending on their age they were given either a feed or sugar water. A baby of three months or older who is capable of going from the last feed through to 6am or 7am should be given sugar water for a week. Once the pattern of once-a-night waking is established, gradually reduce the amount of sugar until he is taking plain water.

This method, along with the routines, will encourage a baby who has suffered from colic and developed the wrong sleep associations to sleep through the night, normally within a couple of weeks. I cannot stress strongly enough that the success of this method very much depends on the use of the sugar water during the first week. Plain water does not have the same success. It is a tip I picked up from an older maternity nurse over 25 years ago and it has never failed me. Parents are often concerned that it will encourage their babies to develop a sweet tooth, or, even worse, rot their teeth. Because of the short period of time the sugar water is used I have never seen any of these problems evolve. I am also pleased to say that my advice has now been backed up by recent research on colic by Dr Peter Lewindon of the Royal Children's Hospital, Brisbane, Australia. Research shows that sugar stimulates the body's natural painkillers and that some babies suffering from colic can be helped by the sugar water solution.

## Crying

I have read in many leading baby books that most young babies cry on average for a total of two hours in a day. This is also the information given by the Thomas Coram Research Unit at London University. They also claim that at six weeks crying reaches a peak, with 25 per cent of babies crying and fussing for at least four hours a day. Dr St James-Roberts also claims that 40 per cent of the crying occurs between 6pm and midnight. Dutch researchers Van de Rijt and Plooij, authors of *Why They Cry: Understanding Child Development in the First Year*, have spent over 20 years studying baby development and they claim that babies become troublesome and demanding when they are going through one of the seven major neurological changes that occur during the first year.

With very young babies I have noticed that they do go through a more unsettled stage around three weeks and six weeks, which tends to coincide with growth spurts. However, I would be absolutely horrified if any of my babies cried for even one hour a day, let alone 2–4 hours! The one thing that parents comment upon time and time again is how happy their baby is on the routine. Of course, my babies do cry; some when they have their nappy changed, others when having their faces washed, and a few try to fight sleep when put in their cots. With the ones that fight sleep, because I know that they are well fed, burped and ready to sleep, I am very strict. I let them fuss and yell for 10–12 minutes until they have settled themselves. This is the only real crying I experience, and even then it is with the minority of my babies and lasts for no longer than a week or two. Understandably, all parents hate to hear their baby cry; many are worried that to put their baby down in a cot to sleep and leave him to cry like this could be psychologically damaging. I would like to reassure you that, provided your baby has been well fed, and that you have followed the routines regarding awake periods and wind-down time, your baby will not suffer psychological damage. In the long term you will have a happy, contented baby who has learned to settle himself to sleep. Many parents who have followed the demand method with the first baby, and my routines with their second baby, would confirm whole-heartedly that my methods are by far the best and, in the long term, the easiest.

Marc Weissbluth MD, Director of the Sleep Disorders Center at the Children's Memorial Hospital, Chicago, says in his book, *Healthy Sleep Habits, Happy Child,* that parents should remember they are *allowing* their baby to cry, not *making* him cry. He also says that it will be much harder for an older baby to learn how to settle himself. Therefore, do not feel guilty or cruel if you have to allow a short spell of crying when your baby is going off to sleep. He will very quickly learn to settle himself, as long as you have made sure he is well fed, and has been awake enough, but not so long that he becomes overtired.

Listed below are the main reasons a healthy baby would cry. Use it as checklist to eliminate the possible cause for your baby crying. At the top of the list is hunger. A tiny baby who is hungry should always be fed, regardless of the routines.

**Hunger**

When your baby is very tiny and fretful and unsettled, it is of course wise to assume that when he cries the problem is hunger and to offer him a feed, even if it is before the time recommended in the routine for his age. One of the main reasons that I find very young breast-fed babies are unsettled in the evening is usually hunger. If your baby feeds well, stays awake for a short spell after feeds, then sleeps well until the next feed, but is unsettled in the evening – it is very possible the cause is hunger. Even if your baby is putting on a good amount of weight each week, you should not rule out hunger. Many mothers I know can produce a lot of milk early on in the day, but come the evening, when tiredness has crept in, the milk supply can decrease dramatically. I would strongly recommend that, for a few nights, you try topping him up with a small amount of expressed milk after his bath. If he settles well then you will know that your milk supply is low at that time of the evening. Please check pages 211 for suggestions on how to deal with this problem.

However, if you find that your baby is unsettled in the evening, or indeed any other time of the day, despite being well fed, it is important that you try to eliminate other reasons for him being fretful. All too often I hear people saying that it is normal for babies to cry a lot in the early days as 'that is what babies do'. During my many years of caring for young babies, I did have some who indeed were very fretful in the early days, no matter what I did to try and help calm them. But I have to stress that out of the hundreds of babies I cared for, there could only have been a handful. If I found that I had a very unsettled baby I would go through every possibility before accepting that there was nothing I could do to help improve things. Babies do have many needs other than feeding, sleeping and being held.

**Tiredness**

Babies under six weeks tend to get tired after one hour of being awake. Although they may not be quite ready to sleep, they need to be kept quiet and calm. Not all babies show obvious sings of tiredness, so, in the early days, after they have been awake for one hour, I would still advise that you take them to their room, so they can wind down gradually. If you can't do that, at least try and keep them in a peaceful part of the house. Try not to allow visitors to overstimulate them during this wind-down period.

**Overtiredness**

No baby under three months should be allowed to stay awake for more than two hours at a time, as they can become very overtired and difficult to settle.

Overtiredness is often a result of overstimulation. An overtired baby reaches a stage where he is unable to drift off to sleep naturally, and the more tired he becomes the more he fights sleep. A baby under three months who is allowed to get into this state, and stays awake for more than two hours, can become almost impossible to settle.

In a situation like this sometimes a short period of 'crying down' has to be used as a last resort to solve the problem. This is the only situation where I would advise that young babies are left to cry for a short period, and even then it can only be done if you are confident that the baby has been well fed and winded.

**Boredom**

Even a newborn baby needs to be awake some of the time. Encourage him to be awake for a short spell after his day feeds Babies under one month love to look at anything black and white, especially pictures of faces, and the ones that fascinate them most will be their faces of their mummy and daddy. Try to divide the toys into ones that are used for wakeful periods and ones that are used for winding-down time. Bright, noisy ones for social time; calm, soothing ones for sleepy times.

**Wind**

All babies take a certain amount of wind while feeding, bottle-fed babies more so than breast-fed ones. Given the opportunity, most babies bring up their wind easily. If you suspect that your baby's crying is caused by wind, check that you are allowing enough time between feeds. I have found overfeeding and demand-feeding to be the main causes of colic in young babies. A breast-fed baby needs at least three hours to digest a full feed, and a formula-fed baby should be allowed three and a half to four hours. This time is always from the beginning of one feed to the beginning of the next feed.

I would also suggest that you keep a close eye on your baby's weight gain. If his weight gain is in excess of 240–300g (8–10oz) a week and he appears to be suffering from wind pains, it could be that he is overfeeding, particularly if he weighs over 3.6kg (8lb) and is feeding two or three times in the night. For details on how to deal with this problem refer to page 69.

### Dummies

The majority of babycare experts frown upon the use of a dummy, claiming that a sucky baby should be allowed to find his thumb. While most very young babies are able to find their thumb, I have yet to see one who can keep it in his mouth long enough to achieve any sucking pleasure. In reality, it takes nearly three months for a baby to develop enough co-ordination to keep his thumb in his mouth for any length of time.

I am amazed how some parents prefer to stick their own fingers in their baby's mouth and spend hour after hour rocking and walking the floor with their baby rather than give him a dummy. They choose to end up with a very demanding baby who refuses to be put down or even to sit for 15 minutes in a baby chair, just because they do not want to give him a dummy.

If used with discretion, I think a dummy can be a great asset, especially for a sucky baby. However, I must stress the importance of never allowing your baby to have the dummy in his cot or allowing him to suck himself to sleep on the dummy. By all means use it to calm him and, if necessary, settle him at sleep times, **but remove it before he falls asleep**. He may yell for a short time but he will soon learn not to expect it while sleeping. Allowing a baby to fall asleep with a dummy in his mouth is one of the worst sleep association problems to solve. He can end up waking several times a night, and each time he will expect the dummy to get back to sleep. This problem can easily be avoided if the dummy is removed just before he drops off to sleep.

I have used dummies with a great number of my babies and have not encountered any serious problems. By being selective in their use, I find that by the age of three months the majority of my babies are rejecting them. If a baby reaches four months and is still using the dummy, I would gradually wean him from it over a period of two weeks; any longer could lead to real attachment problems.

There are two types of dummy available. One has a round cherry-type teat, the other has a flat-shaped teat, which is called an orthodontic teat. Some experts claim that the orthodontic teat shape is better for the baby's mouth, but the problem with this type is that most young babies cannot hold them in for very long. I tend to use the cherry-type teat, and, so far, none of my babies appears to have developed an open bite, which is often the result of a dummy being used excessively once the teeth have come through. Whichever type of dummy you choose, buy several, thus allowing them to be changed frequently. The utmost attention should be paid to cleanliness when using a dummy; it should be washed and sterilised after each use. Never clean it by licking, as one sees so many parents do; there are more germs and bacteria in the mouth than you would believe.

## Hiccups

Hiccups are very normal among tiny babies, and very few get distressed by them. Hiccups often happen after a feed. If it has been a night-time feed and your baby is due to go down for a sleep, it is advisable to go ahead and put him down regardless. If you wait until the hiccups are finished, there is a bigger chance of him falling asleep in your arms, which is something to be avoided at all costs. If your baby is one of the rare ones who gets upset by their hiccups, then try giving him the recommended dose of gripe water, which can sometimes help.

### Possetting

It is very common for some babies to bring up a small amount of milk while being burped or after a feed. It is called possetting, and for most babies it does not create a problem. However, if your baby is regularly gaining more than 240g (8oz) of weight each week it could be that he is drinking too much. With a bottle-fed baby the problem is easily solved as you are able to see how much the baby is drinking and therefore slightly reduce the amount at the feeds during which he appears to possett more. It is more difficult to tell how much a breast-fed baby is drinking. But by keeping a note of which feeds cause more possetting, and reducing the time on the breast at those feeds, the possetting may be reduced.

If your baby is possetting excessively and not gaining weight it could be that he is suffering from a condition called 'reflux' (see below). With babies who are inclined to bring up milk, it is important to keep them as upright as possible after a feed, and special care should be taken when burping.

**Any baby bringing up an entire feed twice in a row should be seen by a doctor immediately.**

### Reflux

Sometimes a baby displaying all the symptoms of colic actually has a condition called gastro-oesophageal reflux. Because the muscle at the lower end of the oesophagus is too weak to keep the milk in the baby's stomach, it comes back up, along with acid from the stomach, causing a very painful burning sensation in the oesophagus. Excessive possetting is one of the symptoms of reflux. However, not all babies with reflux actually sick up the milk, and suffer from what the medical profession call 'silent reflux'. These babies can often be misdiagnosed as having colic. They can be very difficult to feed, constantly arching their backs and screaming during a feed. They also tend to get very irritable when laid flat, and no amount of cuddling or rocking will calm them when they are like this. If your baby displays these symptoms, insist that your doctor does a reflux test. I have seen too many cases of babies being diagnosed as having colic, when in fact they were suffering from reflux, despite not being sick. If you think that your baby is suffering from reflux, it is essential that you do not allow anyone to dismiss the pains as colic. Reflux is very stressful for the baby and parents, and it is essential that you get ongoing advice and support from your GP and health visitor. If you feel that you are not getting the help you need, do not be frightened to ask for a second opinion. If reflux is not the problem, you will at least have eliminated it as a possible cause. If it is the problem, with the help of the right medication, your baby will have been saved months of misery from the pain it can cause. It is important that a baby with reflux is not overfed and is kept as upright as possible during and after feeding. Some babies may need medication for several months until the muscles tighten up. Fortunately, the majority of babies outgrow the condition by the time they are one year old.

## Feeding

### Difficult feeder

The majority of newborn babies take to the breast or bottle quickly and easily. Unlike the new mother, who has much to learn about feeding, the baby instinctively knows what is expected of him. However, there are some babies who, from day one, will fuss and fret within minutes of being put on the breast or being offered the bottle. I often find that some babies who have undergone a particularly hard birth can be more difficult to feed.

If you find that your baby becomes tense and fretful at feed times, try to avoid having visitors then. No matter how well-meaning family and friends may be, it will be impossible to keep things completely calm and quiet if you are having to make conversation. The following guidelines, regardless of whether you are breast- or bottle-feeding, should help make feeding a tense baby easier:

- It is essential that the handling of tense babies is kept to the minimum. Avoid overstimulation and handing the baby from person to person, especially before a feed.
- The feed should be given in a quiet room with a calm atmosphere. Apart from perhaps one person to offer practical help and emotional support, no other person should be allowed in the room.
- Prepare everything needed for the feed well in advance. Try and make sure that you have rested and have eaten.
- Avoid turning on the television during a feed; unplug the telephone and play some calm music while feeding.
- When the baby wakes for his feed, do not change his nappy as this may trigger crying.
- Try swaddling him firmly in a soft cotton sheet to prevent him thrashing his arms and legs around. Make sure that you are comfortable before you start feeding.
- Do not attempt to latch the baby on to the breast or put the bottle straight in his mouth if he is crying. Hold him firmly in the feeding position and calm him down with continuous gentle patting on the back.
- Try holding a dummy in his mouth. Once he has calmed down and has sucked steadily for a few minutes, then very quickly ease the dummy out and offer him the breast or the bottle.

If your baby has been feeding well and suddenly starts to refuse the breast or bottle, it could be because he is feeling unwell. Ear infections can easily go undetected and are a very common cause of a baby not wanting to feed. If your baby shows any of the following signs it would be advisable to consult your doctor:

- Sudden loss of appetite, and becoming upset when offered a feed.
- Disruption to the normal sleep pattern.

- Suddenly becoming clingy and whingy.
- Becomes lethargic and unsociable.

## Excessive night feeding

I have found that all babies, even demand-fed babies, are capable of sleeping one longer spell between feeds by the time they reach 4–6 weeks of age. Beatrice Hollyer and Lucy Smith, authors of an excellent book called *Sleep: the Secret of Problem-free Nights*, describe this longer stretch of sleep as the 'core night' and I have referred to it on page 133. They advise parents to take their cue from this, which they believe is the foundation of encouraging a baby to sleep right through the night.

I believe that by the end of the second week a baby who weighed 2.1kg (7lb) or more at birth should really only need one feed in the night (between midnight and 6am). This is provided, of course, that he is feeding well at all of his daytime feeds and gets a full feed between 10pm and 11pm. In my experience, regardless of whether they are breast- or bottle-fed, a baby who continues to feed two or three times in the night will eventually begin to cut back on his daytime feeds. A vicious circle soon emerges, where the baby ends up genuinely needing to feed in the night so that his daily nutritional needs can be met.

With bottle-fed babies it is easier to avoid a pattern of excessive night time feeding evolving by monitoring the amounts they are getting during the day. The chart on page 63 gives details of how much milk a formula-fed baby would need to satisfy his daily nutritional needs during the first month. Following these guidelines, as well as the core night suggestions (page 207), will prevent excessive night feeding for a formula-fed baby.

Excessive night-time feeding is considered normal for breast-fed babies and is actually encouraged by many breast-feeding experts. Mothers are advised to have their baby sleep with them, so that he can feed on and off throughout the night.

Much emphasis is placed on the fact that the hormone prolactin, which is necessary for making breast milk, is produced more at night. The theory is that mothers who feed their babies more in the night than in the day are much more likely to sustain a good milk supply. This advice obviously works for some mothers, but breast-feeding statistics prove that it clearly doesn't for many others, as so many give up in the first month. As I've said, I believe that the exhaustion caused by so many night-time feeds is one of the main reasons that so many mothers give up breast-feeding.

In my experience from working with hundreds of breast-feeding mothers, I have found that a good stretch of sleep in the night results in the breasts producing more milk. A full and satisfying feed in the middle of the night will ensure that the baby settles back to sleep quickly until the morning.

The following guidelines give the main causes of excessive night-time feeding and how it can be avoided:

- A premature baby or a very tiny baby would need to feed more often than three-hourly, and medical advice should be sought on how best to deal with these special circumstances.
- If he feeds well at every feed (a baby over 3.6kg (8lb) should always be offered the second breast) and is sleeping well at all the other sleep times, he may not be getting enough from the 10.30pm feed.
- If a low milk supply at the last feed is the problem, it can easily be solved by ensuring your baby takes a full feed from a bottle of either formula or expressed milk. If you decide to offer expressed milk, you will need to allow enough time to express for the feed, which can be added to milk from the morning expressing.
- Many women are concerned that introducing a bottle too early may reduce the baby's desire to take the breast. All of my babies are offered one bottle a day as a matter of course and I have never had one baby who had nipple confusion or refused the breast. It has the added advantage that the father can give the last feed and enable the mother to get to bed by 10pm.

- If after one week of giving a full feed at this time there is no improvement, and your baby still is waking several times a night, it is more likely that your baby has a problem with his sleeping than with his feeding. I suggest that you continue to offer the bottle for a further week and refer to page 223 for more advice on night waking.
- Babies under 3.6kg (8lb) in weight who are changed to the second breast before reaching the fatty, rich hind milk in the first breast will be more likely to wake more than once in the night.
- If a baby weighs over 3.6kg (8lb) in weight at birth and is only feeding from one breast at a feed, then he may not be getting enough milk, and should be offered the second breast at some or all of his feeds. If he has fed for 20–25 minutes on the first breast then try to get him to take 5–10 minutes from the second. If he refuses, try waiting 15–20 minutes before offering it again.

The majority of the babies on my routines who are only feeding once in the night gradually push themselves right through the night, dropping the middle-of-the-night feed as soon as they are physically capable. However, occasionally I get a baby who reaches six weeks and continues to wake at 2am looking for a feed. In my experience, allowing these babies to continue to feed at this time usually results in them reducing the amount they take at 7am, often cutting this feed out altogether. When this happens, I would use the core night method to ensure that when the baby is ready to reduce the number of feeds he is having over a 24-hour period, it is always the middle-of-the-night feed that he drops first.

**The core night**

The core night method has been used for many years by maternity nurses and parents who believe in routine. It works on the principle that once a baby sleeps for one longer spell in the night, he should never again be fed during the hours slept in the course of the core night. If he wakes during those hours, he should be left for a few minutes to settle himself back to sleep. If he refuses to settle, then other methods apart from feeding should be used to settle him. Hollyer and Smith recommend patting, offering a dummy or giving a sip of water. Attention should be kept to the minimum while reassuring the baby that you are there. They claim that following this approach will, within days, have your baby sleeping at least the hours of his first core night. It also teaches the baby the most important of two sleep skills: how to go to sleep, and how to go back to sleep after surfacing from a non-REM (rapid eye movement) sleep.

Dr Brian Symon, author of *Silent Nights* and a senior lecturer in general practice at the University of Adelaide, recommends a similar approach for babies over six weeks. Babies who are putting on a good amount of weight each week, but who are still waking at 3am should be offered the dummy or some cool boiled water. If the baby refuses to settle then give the shortest feed possible that will allow him to settle.

Neither of these methods of dealing with night feeding are new. Babycare expert Christine Bruell, who has advised over 35,000 mothers during her 40-year career, also advises offering cool boiled water to a thriving baby over four weeks of age if he keeps regularly waking at 2am.

Before embarking on these methods, the following points should be read carefully to make sure that your baby really is capable of going for a longer spell in the night:

- These methods should never be used with a very small baby or a baby who is not gaining weight. A baby not gaining weight should always be seen by a doctor.
- The above methods should only be used if your baby is regularly gaining 180–240g (6–8oz) each week, and if you are sure that his last feed is substantial enough to help him sleep for the longer stretch in the night.
- The main sign that a baby is ready to cut down on a night feed is a regular weight gain and the reluctance to feed, or feed less, at 7am.

- The aim of using any of the above methods is gradually to increase the length of time your baby can go from his last feed and not to eliminate the night feed in one go.
- The core night method can be used if, over three or four nights, a baby has shown signs that he is capable of sleeping for a longer stretch.
- It can be used to try and reduce the number of times a demand-fed baby is fed in the night and to encourage a longer stretch between feeds, or after his last daytime feed.

### Fussy feeder

If milk feeding is structured properly during the early days of weaning, the majority of babies will happily eat most of the foods they are offered. By the time they reach nine months, babies are expected to be getting most of their nourishment from eating three solid meals a day. Parents are advised to offer their babies a wide variety of foods to ensure they receive all the nutrients they need. However, it is often around this time that many babies start to reject food they have previously enjoyed.

If your baby is between nine and 12 months of age and suddenly starts to reject his food, or becomes fussy and fretful at mealtimes, the following guidelines should help determine the cause:

- Parents often have unrealistic expectations of the amounts of food their baby should have, and serving too large portions can mislead them into thinking that their baby has a feeding problem. The following list, showing the amounts of food a baby aged between nine and 12 months of age needs, will help you decide if your baby is eating enough solids:
  - 3–4 servings of carbohydrate, made up of cereal, wholemeal bread, pasta or potatoes. A serving is one slice of bread, 30g (1oz) of cereal, two tablespoonfuls of pasta, or a small baked potato.
  - 3–4 portions of fruit and vegetables, including raw vegetables. A portion is one small apple, pear or banana, carrot, a couple of cauliflower or broccoli florets, or two tablespoons of chopped green beans.

- ➤ One portion of animal protein or two of vegetable protein. A portion is 30g (1oz) of poultry, meat or fish, or 60g (2oz) of lentil and pulses.

- Self-feeding plays an important role in a baby's mental and physical development as it encourages hand-eye co-ordination and increases his sense of independence. Between six and nine months of age, most babies will start to pick up their food and try to feed themselves. The whole business of feeding can become very messy and mealtimes take much longer. Restricting a baby's natural desire to explore his food and feed himself will only lead to frustration and, very often, refusal to be spoon-fed. Introducing lots of finger foods and allowing him to eat part of his meal by himself, regardless of the mess he makes, will make him much more inclined to take the remainder from you off a spoon.
- By the time a baby reaches nine months of age, he will become more interested in the colour, shape and texture of his food. A baby who is still having all the different foods mashed up together will quickly begin to get bored with even his favourite foods and this is one of the main reasons that babies lose interest in vegetables.
- Offering your baby a selection of vegetables of various textures and colours at each meal in small amounts will be more appealing to him than a large amount of just one or two vegetables.
- Sweet puddings and ice cream desserts served on a regular basis are major causes of babies and toddlers refusing their main course. Even babies as young as nine months can quickly learn that if they refuse the savoury foods and fuss enough, they will more than likely be given the pudding. It is better to restrict puddings and desserts to special occasions, and serve your baby fresh fruit, yoghurt or cheese as a second course.
- If your baby rejects a particular food, it is important that he should be offered it again a couple of weeks later. Babies' likes and dislikes regarding food fluctuate a good deal in the first year and parents who fail to keep reintroducing food

that is rejected usually find that their baby ends up eating a very restricted diet.

- Giving large amounts of juice or water prior to a meal can result in a baby not eating very well. Try to offer him drinks midway between meals, not an hour before. Also, at mealtimes encourage him to eat at least half of the solids before offering him a drink of water or well-diluted juice.
- The timing of meals also plays a big part in how well a baby eats. A baby who is having his breakfast solids later than 8am is unlikely to be very hungry for his lunch much before 1pm. Likewise, a baby who is having teatime solids later than 5pm may be getting too tired to eat well.
- Giving too many snacks in between meals, especially hard-to-digest foods like bananas or cheese, can often take the edge off a baby's appetite. Try restricting snacks for a couple of days to see if his appetite improves at mealtimes.

If you are concerned that your baby is not taking enough solids, it is advisable to seek advice from your health visitor or doctor. Keeping a diary for a week, listing the times and amounts of all food and drinks consumed, will help them to determine the cause of your baby's feeding problems.

### Low milk supply

As they grow, all babies will increase the amount they drink. However, the feeds must be structured to co-ordinate with the baby's growth, thereby encouraging him to take more milk at individual feeds. If not, he will be very likely to continue to feed little and often.

All too often, I get calls from the parents of older babies who are still following the demand rules of milk feeding. While the majority of these babies are over 12 weeks and are physically capable of drinking more at individual feeds, they continue to feed as they did as newborns – often 8–10 times a day.

Many breast-fed babies are still having only one breast at each feed, while bottle-fed babies may only be taking 90–120ml

(3–4oz) of formula. In order to go for longer spells between feeds, these babies should be taking from both breasts at each feed, or have a formula feed of 210–240ml (7–8oz). It is my firm belief that it is during those early days of milk feeding that the foundation is laid for healthy eating habits in the future. To avoid long-term feeding problems that can affect your baby's sleep, it is advisable to structure and solve any milk-feeding problems early on.

Not producing enough milk, especially later in the day, is a very common problem for breast-feeding mothers and one of the major reasons breast-feeding goes wrong. I believe that hunger is why so many babies are fretful and difficult to settle in the evening. If the problem of a low milk supply is not resolved in the early days, then a pattern soon emerges of the baby needing to feed on and off all evening to try and satisfy his needs. Mothers are advised that this constant feeding is normal and the best way to increase the milk supply, but in my experience, it usually has the opposite effect. Because the amount of milk the breasts produce is dictated by the amount of milk the baby drinks, these frequent feeds signal the breasts to produce milk little and often. These small feeds will rarely satisfy the baby, leaving him hungry and irritable.

I believe that the stress involved in frequently feeding a very hungry, irritable and often overtired baby can cause many mothers to become so exhausted that their milk supply is reduced even further. Exhaustion and a low milk supply go hand in hand. I am convinced that by expressing a small amount of milk during the early weeks of breast-feeding, when the breasts are producing more milk than the baby needs, the mother can help avoid the problem of a low milk supply.

If your baby is under one month of age and not settling in the evening, it is possible the cause is a low milk supply. Expressing at the times suggested in the routine below should help solve this problem. The short amount of time you spend expressing will ensure that during any future growth spurts you will be producing enough milk to meet any increase in your baby's appetite. If your baby is over one month and not settling in the evening or after daytime feeds, the following six-day plan will quickly help to increase your milk supply. The temporary introduction of top-up feeds will ensure that your baby is not subjected to hours of irritability and anxiety caused by hunger, which is what usually happens when mothers resort to demand-feeding to increase their milk supply.

## Plan for increased milk supply

### Days one to three

**6.45am**

- Express 30ml (1oz) from each breast.
- Baby should be awake, and feeding no later than 7am, regardless of how often he fed in the night.
- He should be offered 20–25 minutes on the fullest breast, then 10–15 minutes on the second breast.
- Do not feed after 7.45am. He can stay awake for up to two hours.

**8am**

- It is very important that you have a breakfast of cereal, toast and a drink no later than 8am.

**9am**

- If your baby has not been settling well for his nap, offer him 5–10 minutes on the breast from which he last fed.
- Try to have a short rest when the baby is sleeping.

**10am**

- **Baby must be fully awake now, regardless of how long he slept.**
- He should be given 20–25 minutes from the breast he last fed on while you drink a glass of water and have a small snack.
- Express 60ml (2oz) from the second breast, then offer him 10–20 minutes on the same breast.

**11.45am**

- He should be given the 60ml (2oz) that you expressed to ensure that he does not wake up hungry during his midday nap.
- It is very important that you have a good lunch and a rest before the next feed.

**2pm**

- **Baby should be awake and feeding no later than 2pm, regardless of how long he has slept.**
- Give him 20–25 minutes from the breast he last fed on while you drink a glass of water. Express 60ml (2oz) from the second breast, then offer 10–20 minutes on the same breast.

**4pm**

- Baby will need a short nap according to the routine appropriate for his age.

**5pm**

- **Baby should be fully awake and feeding no later than 5pm.**
- Give 15–20 minutes from both breasts.

**6.15pm**

- Baby should be offered a top-up feed of expressed milk from the bottle. A baby under 3.6kg (8lb) in weight will probably settle with 60–90ml (2–3oz); bigger babies may need 120–150ml (4–5oz).
- Once your baby is settled, it is important that you have a good meal and a rest.

**8pm**

- Express from both breasts.

**10pm**

- It is important that you express from both breasts at this time, as the amount you get will be a good indicator of how much milk you are producing.

- Arrange for your husband or another family member to give the 10.30pm feed to the baby so you can have an early night.

**10.30pm**

- Baby should be awake and feeding no later than 10.30pm. He can be given a full feed of either formula or expressed milk from a bottle. Refer to the chart on page 63 for details of the amounts to give.

**In the night**

A baby who has had a full feed from the bottle at 10.30pm should manage to get to 2–2.30am. He should then be offered 20–25 minutes from the first breast, then 10–15 minutes from the second. In order to avoid a second waking in the night at 5am, it is very important that he feeds from both breasts.

If your baby fed well at 10.30pm and wakes earlier than 2am, the cause may not be hunger. The following checklist gives other reasons which may be causing him to wake earlier:

- Kicking off the covers may be the cause of your baby waking earlier than 2am. A baby under six weeks who wakes up thrashing around may still need to be fully swaddled. A baby over six weeks may benefit from being half-swaddled under the arms in a thin cotton sheet. With all babies, it is important to ensure that the top sheet is tucked in well, down the sides and at the bottom of the cot.
- The baby should be fully awake at the 10.30pm feed. With a baby who is waking up before 2am, it may be worthwhile keeping him awake longer, and offering him some more milk just before you settle him at around 11.15pm.

**Day four**

By day four, your breasts should be feeling fuller in the morning and the following alterations should be made to the above plan:

- If your baby is sleeping well between 9am and 9.45am, reduce the time on the breast at 9am to five minutes.
- The top-up at 11.45am can be reduced by 30ml (1oz) if he is

sleeping well at lunchtime, or shows signs of not feeding so well at the 2pm feed.

- The expressing at the 2pm feed should be dropped, which should mean that your breasts are fuller by the 5pm feed.
- If you feel your breasts are fuller at 5pm, make sure he totally empties the first breast before putting him on to the second breast. If he has not emptied the second breast before the bath, he should be offered it again after the bath, and before he is given a top-up.
- The 8pm expressing should be dropped and the 10pm expressing brought forward to 9.30pm. It is important that both breasts are completely emptied at the 9.30pm expressing.

**Day five**

- Dropping the 2pm and 8pm expressing on the fourth day should result in your breasts being very engorged on the morning of the fifth day; it is very important that the extra milk is totally emptied at the first feed in the morning.
- At the 7am feed the baby should be offered 20–25 minutes on the fullest breast, then 10–15 minutes on the second breast, after you have expressed. The amount you express will depend on the weight of your baby. It is important that you take just the right amount so that enough is left for your baby to get a full feed. If you managed to express a minimum of 120ml (4oz) at the 10pm feed, you should manage to express the following amounts:

    (a) Baby weighing 3.6–4.5kg (8–10lb) – express 120ml (4oz)
    (b) Baby weighing 4.5–5.4kg (10–12lb) – express 90ml (3oz)
    (c) Baby weighing over 5.4kg (12lb) – express 60ml (2oz)

**Day six**

By the sixth day, your milk supply should have increased enough for you to drop all top-up feeds, and follow the breast-feeding routines appropriate for your baby's age laid out in Chapter 6. It is very important that you also follow the guidelines for expressing as set out in the routines. This will ensure that you will be able to satisfy your baby's increased appetite during his next growth spurt. I would also suggest that you continue with one bottle of either expressed or formula milk at the 10.30pm feed until your baby is weaned on to solids at six months. This will allow the feed to be given by your husband or partner, enabling you to get to bed earlier after you have expressed, which, in turn, will make it easier for you to cope with the middle-of-the-night feed.

### Refusal of milk

The amount of milk a six-month-old baby drinks will gradually begin to reduce as his intake of solid food increases. However, up to the age of nine months, a baby still needs a minimum of 500–600ml (17–20oz) a day of breast or formula milk. This daily amount gradually reduces to a minimum of 350ml (12oz) at one year of age. If your baby is losing interest or refusing some of his milk feeds and taking less than the recommended amounts, careful attention should be given to the timing of solids and the type of food given.

The following guidelines will help you determine the cause of your baby refusing his milk feeds:

- Up to the age of six months, a baby should still be taking 4–5 full milk feeds morning and evening. A full milk feed consists of 210–240ml (7–8oz) or a feed from both breasts. Babies under six months who are weaned early on the advice of a health visitor or GP should not be given solids in the middle of their milk feed. They will be more likely to refuse the remainder of their formula or the second breast. Give most of the milk feed first, then the solids.
- A baby under six months of age still needs a full milk feed at 11am, even if he is being weaned early on medical advice. Introducing breakfast too soon or offering too much solid food first thing in the morning can cause a baby to cut down too quickly or to refuse the 11am feed.
- The 11am milk feed should be reduced and eliminated between the ages of six and seven months.

- Giving lunchtime solids at 2pm and evening solids at 5pm is the reason many babies under seven months cut down too quickly or refuse their 6pm milk feed. Until he is used to solids, it is better to give a baby his lunchtime solids at 11am and his evening solids after he has had a full milk feed at 6pm.
- Giving hard-to-digest foods such as banana or avocado at the wrong time of the day can cause a baby to cut back on the next milk feed. Until a baby reaches seven months, it is better to serve these types of food after the 6pm feed, rather than during the day.
- Babies over six months of age who begin to refuse milk are often being allowed too many snacks in between meals or too much juice. Try replacing juice with water and cutting out snacks in between meals.
- Between nine and 12 months, some babies begin refusing the bedtime milk feed, which is a sign that they are ready to drop their third milk feed. If this happens, it is important to reduce the amount given at the 2.30pm feed, before eventually dropping it altogether.

### Refusal of solids

With babies of six months or older, the refusal of solids often occurs because they drink too much milk, especially if they are still feeding in the middle of the night. Every day I speak to parents of babies and toddlers who will barely touch solids, let alone eat three meals a day. In the majority of these cases, the babies are still being milk-fed on demand, some feeding as often as two or three times in the night. While milk is still a very important food for babies at six months, failing to structure the time of milk feeds and the amounts given can seriously affect the introduction of solids. If your baby is refusing solids, the following guidelines will help you determine the cause:

- The recommended age to introduce solids is at six months. If your baby is six months and sleeping through the night from 10pm this feed should gradually be reduced and eliminated.

- A baby is ready to be weaned when he shows signs that his appetite is no longer satisfied with 4–5 full milk feeds a day. A full milk feed is either a formula-feed of 240ml (8oz) or a feed from both breasts. See page 166 for signs that your baby is ready for weaning.
- If your baby reaches six months and is having more than 4–5 full milk feeds a day, his refusal of solids may be caused by drinking too much milk. It is important to cut right back on his 11am milk feed to encourage him to eat more solids at that time. By the end of six months, a baby's milk intake should be around 600ml (20oz) a day, divided between three drinks a day and small amounts used in food. If your baby is still refusing solids at this age, despite cutting down on his milk intake, it is important that you discuss the problem as soon as possible with your doctor or health visitor.

## Sleepy feeder

Sometimes a very sleepy baby may be inclined to keep dozing during the feed, but if he does not want to take the required amount he will end up wanting to feed again in an hour or two. This is a good time to change his nappy, burp him and encourage him to finish his feed. Making a little effort in the early days to keep your baby awake enough to drink the correct amount at each feed, and at the times given in the routine, will in the long term be well worthwhile. Some babies will take half the feed, have a stretch and kick for 10–15 minutes, and then be happy to take the rest. The important thing that I have found with sleepy babies was not to force them to stay awake by talking too much or jiggling them about. By putting your baby under the playgym or cot mobile and leaving him for 10 minutes, you will probably find that he will get enough of a second wind to take more of a feed. During the first months, allow up to 45 minutes to one hour for a feed.

Obviously, if he does not feed well at a particular feed, and wakes early from his sleep, he must be fed. Do not attempt to try and stretch him to the next feed, otherwise he will be so tired that the next feed will also become another sleepy feed. Top him up and treat the feed like a night feed, and try to settle him back to sleep so that you can get his feeding back on track for the evening.

## Sleeping

### Difficulties in settling

If your baby is difficult to settle at nap times, it is essential that you pay particular attention to the time you begin settling him and how long you spend trying to do this. With the majority of babies, the main reason they are hard to settle is overtiredness or overstimulation. Once you are confident that you have your baby's feeding and sleeping on track, I would strongly advise you to help your baby learn how to settle himself to sleep. Although it will be very difficult to listen to him cry, he will very quickly learn how to go to sleep by himself. He should never be left for more than 5–10 minutes before being checked. From my experience in helping hundreds of parents with babies who have had serious sleeping problems, once a baby learns how to settle himself, he becomes happier and more relaxed. Once proper daytime sleep is established, night-time sleep will also improve.

The following guidelines should help your baby learn how to settle himself:

- A baby who is allowed to fall asleep on the breast or bottle and is then put in the cot will be more likely to have disruptive nap times. When he comes into a light sleep 30–45 minutes after falling asleep, he will be less likely to settle himself back to sleep without your help. If your baby falls asleep while feeding, put him on the changing mat and rearrange his nappy. This should rouse him enough to go down in the cot semi-awake.
- Overtiredness is a major cause of babies not settling and not

sleeping well during the day. A baby under three months who is allowed to stay awake for longer than two hours at a time may get so overtired that he goes on to fight sleep for a further two hours. After three months, the majority of babies, as they get older, will manage to stay awake slightly longer, sometimes up to two and a half hours at a time. A close eye should be kept on all babies after they have been awake for one and a half hours so that you do not miss the cue for sleep.

- Overhandling prior to sleep time is another major problem with young babies. Everyone wants just one little cuddle. Unfortunately, several little cuddles add up and can leave the baby fretful, overtired and difficult to settle. Your baby is not a toy. Do not feel guilty about restricting the handling in the early weeks, especially prior to sleep time.
- Overstimulation before sleep time is another major cause of babies not settling well. Babies under six months should be allowed a quiet wind-down time of 20 minutes before being put down to sleep. With babies over six months, avoid games and activities that cause them to get overexcited. With all babies, regardless of age, avoid excessive talking at put-down time. Talk quietly and calmly using the same simple phrases: 'Night-night, teddy. Night-night, dolly. Sweet dreams.' Once you leave the room do not keep going back to check.
- The wrong sleep association can also cause long-term sleep problems. It is essential that a baby goes down in his cot awake and learns to settle himself. For a baby who has already learned the wrong sleep associations, this problem can rarely be solved without some amount of crying. Fortunately, the majority of babies, if they are allowed, will learn to settle themselves within a few days.

### Early-morning waking

All babies and young children come into a light sleep between 5am and 6am. Some will settle back to sleep for a further hour or so but many do not. I believe there are two things that determine whether a baby will become an earlier riser. One is the darkness of the nursery. It would be an understatement to say I am obsessed with how dark the nursery should be, but I am totally convinced that it is the reason the majority of my babies quickly resettle themselves to sleep when they come into a light sleep at 5–6am. Once the nursery door is shut and the curtains drawn, it should be so dark that not even the faintest trace of toys or books can be seen. A glimpse of these things will be enough to fully waken a baby from a drowsy state and make him want to start the day.

How parents deal with early wakings during the first three months will also determine whether their baby will become a child who is an early riser. During the first few weeks, a baby who is waking and feeding at 2–2.30am may wake around 6am and genuinely need to feed. However, it is essential to treat this feed like a night-time feed. It should be done as quickly and quietly as possible with the use of only a small night-light and without talking or eye contact. The baby should then be settled back to sleep until 7–7.30am. If possible, avoid changing the nappy as this usually wakes the baby too much.

Once the baby is sleeping and feeding nearer 4am, waking at 6am is not usually related to hunger. This is the one and only time I would advise parents to help their baby return to sleep. At this stage the most important thing is to get him back to sleep quickly, even if it means cuddling him and offering him a dummy until 7am. Listed below are guidelines that will help your baby not to become an early riser:

- Avoid using a night-light or leaving the door open once you have put him down to sleep. Research shows that chemicals in the brain work differently in the dark, preparing it for sleep. Even the smallest chink of light can be enough to awaken the baby fully when he enters his light sleep.
- Kicking off the bedcovers can also cause babies under six months to wake early. In my experience, all babies under this age sleep better if tucked in securely. The sheet needs to be

placed lengthways across the width of the cot to ensure that a minimum of 20cm (8in) is tucked in at the far side and a minimum of 10cm (4in) at the near side. I would also advise rolling up a small hand towel and pushing it down between the spars and the mattress at the near side.

- Babies who work their way up the cot and get out of the covers will benefit from being put in a lightweight 100 per cent cotton sleeping bag and tucked in with a sheet as described above. Depending on the weather, blankets may not be necessary.
- Once a baby starts to move around the cot and is capable of rolling, I would advise that you remove the sheets and blankets and use only the sleeping bag. This will allow your baby to move around unrestricted, without the worry that he might get cold in the middle of the night. It is important to choose a sleeping bag that is suitable for the time of year.
- Do not drop the 10.30pm feed until your baby has reached six months and has started solids. If he goes through a growth spurt before he starts solids, he can be offered extra milk at this time. This reduces the chances of waking early due to hunger, which can occur if the 10.30pm feed is dropped too soon.
- A baby who is over six months and has dropped the 10.30pm feed should be encouraged to stay awake until 7pm. If he is falling into a deep sleep before this time, he will be much more likely to wake before 7am.

## Excessive night waking

Until the mother's milk comes in, a newborn baby may wake and need to be fed several times a night. By the end of the first week, a baby who weighs over 3.2kg (7lb) should manage to sleep for a stretch of four hours from the 10–11pm feed, provided his feeding needs are being fully met during the day. Smaller babies may still need to feed three-hourly around the clock. In my experience, all babies who are healthy and well fed will, between four and six weeks of age, manage to sleep one longer spell of 5–6 hours. By following my routines this longer spell should happen in the night. The main aim of my routines is to help parents structure their baby's feeding and sleeping needs during the day so as to avoid excessive night waking.

How long a baby will continue to wake for a feed in the night depends very much on the individual baby. Some babies between six and eight weeks sleep through after the 10.30pm feed, others between 10 and 12 weeks. Some may even take longer. All babies will sleep through the night as soon as they are physically and mentally able, provided the daytime feeding and sleeping is being properly structured. Listed below are the main causes of excessive night-time waking in healthy babies under one year old:

- Sleeping too much during the day. Even very small babies need to be awake some of the time. The baby should be encouraged to stay awake for one to one and a half hours after daytime feeds. Between six and eight weeks most babies are capable of staying awake for up to two hours.
- Not feeding enough during the day. If excessive night feeding is to be avoided, the baby needs to have six feeds between 7am and 11pm. To fit in this number of feeds, the day must start at 7am.
- Not feeding enough at each feed. In the early days a baby needs a minimum of 25 minutes on one breast. A baby who weighs over 3.6kg (8lb) should be offered the second breast.
- Breast-fed babies will be more likely to wake several times a night if they do not get enough to eat at the 10.30pm feed and may need a top-up after this feed.
- Babies under six weeks have a very strong Moro reflex (see page 83) and can wake themselves several times a night by the sudden startle and jerk. These babies will benefit from being swaddled in a lightweight stretch cotton sheet.
- Older babies often wake several times at night because they have kicked their covers off and are cold, or they may have got their legs caught between the spars of the cot. A sleeping bag will help them avoid becoming cold and will prevent

them from getting their legs caught in the spars.

- The baby has learned the wrong sleep associations. Between two and three months his sleep cycle changes and he will come into a light sleep several times at night. If the baby is used to being fed, rocked or given a dummy to get to sleep, he will need the same assistance to resettle himself in the night.
- Parents who leave the nursery door open or leave on a night-light are more likely to be woken several times a night.
- If the baby's milk feeds are reduced too quickly when solids are introduced, he will begin to wake in the night genuinely needing a milk feed.

### Illness – the effect on sleep

The majority of my first babies manage to get through the first year without suffering the usual colds and coughs that seem to plague my second and third babies. By the time most first babies I have cared for experience a cold, their sleep is so well established that wakings in the night are very rare. With second and third babies this is not the case as they usually catch their first cold at a much younger age from a brother or sister and disrupted nights are inevitable. A baby under three months of age will usually need help to get through the night when they have a cold or are ill. A young baby with a cold can get very distressed, especially when he is feeding, as he will not have learned to breathe through his mouth.

When a sick baby needs attention in the evening and during the night it should be given calmly and quietly. I believe that a sick baby needs more rest than a healthy baby. Lots of visitors and activity in the nursery during the evening and in the night should be avoided. When I have had to care for a sick baby who wakes several times at night I find it less disruptive if I sleep in the same room as the baby. It enables me to attend to him quickly and I am less likely to interrupt the sleep of elder siblings by to-ing and fro-ing along the corridor.

Occasionally, I find that an older baby who has dropped

night-time feeds will, once he has recovered, continue to wake up in the night looking for the same attention he received when he was unwell. For the first few nights I would check him and offer him some cool boiled water, but once I was convinced he was totally recovered, I would get tough and leave him to settle himself. In my experience, parents who are not prepared to do this usually end up with a baby who develops a long-term sleep problem.

If your baby develops a cold or cough, regardless of how mild it appears, he should be seen by a doctor. All too often I hear from distressed parents of babies with serious chest infections, which could possibly have been avoided if they had been seen by a doctor earlier. Too many mothers delay taking their baby to the doctor, worried that they will be classed as neurotic, but it is important that you discuss with your doctor any concerns you have about your baby's health, however small. If your baby is ill, it is essential that you follow your doctor's advice to the letter, especially on feeding.

### The lunchtime nap

The lunchtime nap is a fundamental part of my CLB routines. Recent research shows that children up to the age of two years benefit physically and psychologically from a proper, structured nap in the middle of the day. As your baby grows and is more active, this nap will become his time to rest and recover from the morning's activities and will enable him to enjoy his afternoons with you and others.

Like many aspects of the routines, it takes time to establish and you will need to be patient and persevere until your baby learns the habit. Once it is in place this nap will not only be of enormous value to your baby, but also to you. Many of the mothers I have worked with over the years have told me how much of a lifesaver this lunchtime nap is. In the early months you can use it to have some much-needed rest yourself. Once your baby sleeps through the night it can be the time you catch up on housework or phone calls – or even some work, as many mums testify. This nap can continue well into the second year and even into the third for some toddlers. If you have another baby while your toddler still enjoys a lunchtime nap, this will be invaluable.

In the early days a lunchtime nap may sometimes go wrong and your baby will refuse to go back to sleep, even when offered a feed. The baby comes into a light sleep, usually 30–45 minutes after he has gone to sleep. Some babies will wake up fully and it is important that they learn how to settle themselves if the wrong sleep associations are to be avoided.

## Sleep associations

During the early months many babies are happy to doze on and off in a car seat or Moses basket, which can be convenient as it allows parents more flexibility. Unfortunately, once the baby becomes bigger and more active, he is unlikely to continue to sleep well or for long enough in the car seat. If this habit is established it can be very difficult to get him to sleep in his cot during the day. The sleep in the car seat is unlikely to be satisfying and, as he gets older, he will most likely spend the time catnapping and become tired and irritable later on. The knock-on effect of this is that he might not feed well at teatime or fall asleep before he's had all of his bedtime milk. Night wakings due to hunger can then result, leaving all of you tired the next day and so the problem continues to get worse. You need to start putting him down for this sleep in his cot, in the dark, as early as possible. If this isn't possible because of older children and school runs, try to settle the baby in his pram or buggy in a quieter part of the house so he gets as much undisturbed sleep as he can.

If sleep associations have taken root, you will need to focus on getting him to sleep during this nap period whatever it takes. This is known as *assisting the baby to sleep*. Take him out in the buggy or the car, or into bed or on to the sofa with you, and let him have the two hours he needs. I usually found that if I did this for a week or even 10 days, the baby's sleep cycle would adapt to it and it was easier then to put him down in his cot with just a little bit of 'crying down'.

### Hunger

Babies who start weaning nearer six months might need more solids or more milk. A baby up to the age of nine months needs a minimum of 600ml (20oz) milk every day. Once he reaches nine months he still needs 500–600ml (17–20oz) a day. By seven months he should be eating three meals a day and solids should be well established. Check *The Contented Little Baby Book of Weaning* for the recommended amounts. If you have weaned at six months you will need to move through the guide quickly to build up the right amounts of food.

Small babies can have their 11am feed brought forward to 10.30am so that you can split the feed and give them a top-up just before they go down for the nap. This way you can be sure they are not hungry as they go down.

Older babies should have lunch at 11am. You can go back to topping him up just before he goes down with some of his 2.30pm feed – try this for a week and see if it helps. If it's obvious after a week that hunger is the problem you need to increase his solids throughout the day, bring lunch back to the correct time and then drop the top-up. Do this gradually over the course of another week.

If solids are well established and the baby is no longer having milk at this feed, he still needs to have a good drink of water or well-diluted juice with his lunch, as well as a drink mid-morning. Thirst can be a reason why a baby wakes from his nap, especially during hot weather.

### Daytime sleep

Look at his morning nap and check that he is having the right amounts at the right times. Try to ensure that it is not before 9am for young babies and not before 9.15–9.30am for older babies. If you find he is sleeping too long at this nap it could well be the reason for him not sleeping so long at lunchtime.

The lunchtime nap is ultimately the more important nap as it is longer and fits in with a baby's natural sleep cycles. Somewhere between nine and 12 months the majority of babies need to cut back on this nap and some may want to cut it out altogether, especially if they are sleeping until 7.30–7.45am. Other babies may just need 10–15 minutes' catnapping. To reduce the morning nap, try cutting it back by 10 minutes every three or four days until a baby under nine months is having only 20–25 minutes. You might have to move lunch forward if he is getting tired, and put him down earlier for his nap.

### What to do when it goes wrong

Your baby won't be able to make it through the afternoon if he's only had 40–60 minutes' sleep at lunchtime. I find the best way to deal with this is to allow him 30 minutes more sleep after the 2.30pm feed and then a further 30 minutes at 4.30pm. This should stop him getting overtired and irritable, and you can get back on track again at 5pm and ensure he goes down well at 7pm. If a very young baby has slept between 3–4pm on the school run he might be ready to sleep at 6pm. With a young baby you just have to accept this. I suggest that you bring the 5pm feed forward to 4.30pm and have him in bed for 6pm. An older baby might make it to 6.15–6.30pm and you will need to bring tea and bathtime forward appropriately. As the baby gets older he will be able to manage without an afternoon nap and you can get back to putting him down at 7pm, provided his lunchtime sleep has been long enough.

If you 'tweak' the routines to allow him more sleep to make up for what he missed at lunchtime you can follow my recommendations at the beginning of each routine for the maximum amount of daily sleep. Always make sure the baby is up and awake by 5pm if you want him to go down well at 7pm.

*Checklist*

- Rule out hunger as the possible reason for waking.

- Check that he is not thirsty by offering him a drink of water just before he goes down.
- Correct any sleep associations, such as falling asleep in the car seat, and ensure he goes down, well fed, in his cot in the dark. Note that it might take some time to get him into good habits, so you will need to be patient.
- Check that the room is really dark and that there are no chinks of light. If a nursery or school run at 12–12.30pm means that baby can't go down in the dark, at least keep him in a quiet section of the house in car seat or pram.
- Eliminate all other reasons for waking, such as noise or not being tucked in properly (remember that the Moro reflex can be very strong in babies under six months so tucking them in securely is very important if they are not to wake themselves up).

When you have checked everything on the list above, and given any changes enough time to work, there may still be a handful of parents who experience problems. These babies will be aged over six months and have serious sleep association problems. Some sleep training may be the only solution in these cases and there are full details of how to approach this in my book, *The Complete Sleep Guide for Contented Babies and Toddlers*. I must stress that this is a last resort and not to be entered into lightly, and certainly not without advice from your doctor or health visitor, who can refer you to a sleep clinic.

### Teething and night waking

In my experience, babies who enjoy a routine from a very early age and have established healthy sleeping habits are rarely bothered by teething. Out of the 300 babies I have helped care for, only a handful have been bothered by teething in the night. In these cases it is usually when the molars come through and then only for a few nights. I have found that babies who wake in the night due to teething are more likely to have suffered from colic and have developed poor sleeping habits.

If your baby is teething and waking in the night but quickly settles back to sleep when given a cuddle or a dummy, teething is probably not the real cause of his waking. A baby who is genuinely bothered by teething pain would be difficult to settle back to sleep. He would also show signs of discomfort during the day, not just at night. I would advise you to check the section on excessive night waking and early-morning waking to eliminate other reasons for your baby waking.

If you are convinced that your baby's night-time wakings are caused by severe teething pain, I suggest you seek advice from your doctor regarding the use of paracetamol. While genuine teething pain may cause a few disruptive nights, it should never last for several weeks. If your baby seems out of sorts, develops a fever and suffers from loss of appetite or diarrhoea, he should be seen by a doctor. Do not assume that these symptoms are just a sign of teething. Very often I have found that what parents thought was teething turned out to be an ear or throat infection.

# Useful addresses

**Black-out lining and roller blinds**
Available from all John Lewis Partnership stores throughout the UK.

**Breast pumps**
Ameda Egnell Ltd
Unit 2, Belvedere Trading Estate
Taunton
Somerset TA1 1BH
Tel: 01823 336362
Fax: 01823 336364

**Baby equipment**
The Great Little Trading Company
Pondwood Close
Moulton Park
Northampton NN3 6DF
Tel: 0870 850 6000
Fax: 01604 640 107
www.gltc.co.uk

**Express Yourself Bras**
www.expressyourselfbras.co.uk

## Organisations

**Foundation for the Study of Infant Deaths**
Artillery House
11–19 Artillery Row
London SW1P 1RT
Tel: 020 7222 8001

**Twins and Multiple Births Association (TAMBA)**
PO Box 30, Little Sutton
South Wirral L66 1TH
Tel: 08707 703305

# Further Reading

*The Complete Sleep Guide for Contented Babies and Todders* by Gina Ford (Vermilion 2006)
*The Contented Child's Food Bible* by Gina Ford (Vermilion 2005)
*The Contented Little Baby Book of Weaning* by Gina Ford (Vermilion 2006)
*The Contented Toddler Years* by Gina Ford (Vermilion 2006)
*The Gina Ford Baby and Toddler Cook Book* by Gina Ford (Vermilion 2005)
*The Great Ormond Street New Baby and Child Care Book* (Vermilion 2004)
*Healthy Sleep Habits, Happy Child* by Marc Weissbluth (Vermilion 2005)
*The New Baby and Toddler Sleep Programme* by Professor John Pearce with Jane Biddler (Vermilion 1999)
*Potty Training in One Week* (Vermilion 2003)
*Remotely Controlled* by Aric Sigman (Vermilion 2005)
*Sleep: The Secret of Problem-free Nights* by Beatrice Hollyer and Lucy Smith (Cassell 2002)
*Solve Your Child's Sleep Problems* by Richard Ferber (Dorling Kindersley 1985)
*What to Expect When You're Breast-feeding . . . And What If You Can't?* by Clare Byam-Cook (Vermilion 2006)
*Your Child's Symptoms Explained* by David Haslam (Vermilion 1997)

# Index

## Also by Gina Ford

## Available from Random House Children's Books

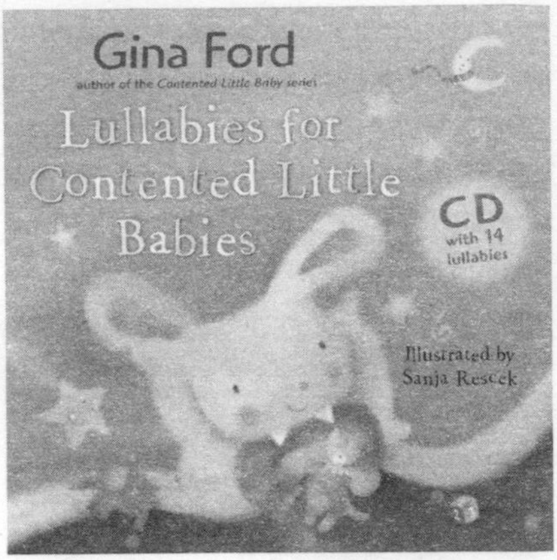


Introducing a brand new, bright and interactive series for babies and toddlers! The Ella and Tom series has been specially created to gently introduce little ones to new experiences and enhance their imaginations.

These touchy feely board books are ideal for babies and parents to share and children will love touching the different textures:

**Ella and Tom: On the Farm**
**Ella and Tom: Let's Play**

Perfect for little hands, these bright lift-the-flap board books encourage learning through play:

**Ella and Tom: Going on a Picnic**
**Ella and Tom: Sleepy Time**

Also available:

**Gina Ford's Bedtime Songs for Contented Little Babies**
A beautiful book of songs and lullabies that will help soothe your baby to sleep. Includes a CD containing over 30 minutes of tranquil songs and music, just right for helping your baby drift off at sleeptime.